Rafaela Maria de Paula Costa
Themis M. Cardinot
Liszt P. de Oliveira

Validation of the Brazilian version of the Hip Outcome Score questionnaire

Rafaela Maria de Paula Costa
Themis M. Cardinot
Liszt P. de Oliveira

Validation of the Brazilian version of the Hip Outcome Score questionnaire

HOS-Brazil

ScienciaScripts

Imprint

Cover image: www.ingimage.com

This book is a translation from the original published under ISBN 978-3-330-76621-1.

Publisher:
Sciencia Scripts
is a trademark of
Dodo Books Indian Ocean Ltd. and OmniScriptum S.R.L publishing group

120 High Road, East Finchley, London, N2 9ED, United Kingdom
Str. Armeneasca 28/1, office 1, Chisinau MD-2012, Republic of Moldova, Europe
Managing Directors: Ieva Konstantinova, Victoria Ursu
info@omniscriptum.com

Printed at: see last page
ISBN: 978-620-8-54061-6

DEDICATORY

To our family and friends for their love and understanding of the time away dedicated to this work.

ACKNOWLEDGEMENTS

To the Orthopaedics Teaching and Assistance Unit of the Pedro Ernesto University Hospital of the State University of Rio de Janeiro, especially the orthopaedic doctors Marcelo Costa de Oliveira Campos and Luiz Otávio Sampaio Penteado and the secretaries Alessandra Messor and Henrique Constantino da Silveira, for their kindness and assistance, and for always being on hand to help.

To the Arthroscopy Laboratory of the Orthopaedics Teaching and Assistance Unit of the Pedro Ernesto University Hospital of the State University of Rio de Janeiro, for the financial support that enabled this work to be carried out.

To the students Nathalia Sundin, Camila de Oliveira, Bernardo Dias and Polyana Noll, for their help in carrying out the fieldwork.

To Lucineide Lima, Juliana Costa and Cíntia Costa for their constant help.

Gustavo Leporace, for his contribution to the statistical analysis.

To the patients who voluntarily agreed to take part in the stages of this work.

SUMMARY

The assessment of quality of life using questionnaires and scales has been used frequently in the healthcare sector to inform patient progress and decide on the most appropriate treatment. Most quality of life assessment and orthopaedic assessment instruments were created in English. For these instruments to be used in a population with a different language and culture to the country where they were developed, it is necessary to follow a number of stages for their translation, cultural adaptation to the language and validation in terms of maintaining the characteristics of the original instrument. The Hip Outcome Score (HOS) is an instrument capable of assessing physically active patients with hip diseases without severe degenerative changes; a condition that other hip assessment instruments are not capable of performing with the same specificity. The stages of translation and cultural adaptation of this questionnaire into Brazilian Portuguese have already been carried out. The aim of this study was to validate the Brazilian version of the HOS questionnaire in a group of physically active patients with a medical diagnosis of femoroacetabular impingement or peritrochanteric pain syndrome. A total of 70 patients were selected, of both genders and aged between 19 and 70 years. The domains studied for the validation process were reliability and validity. These domains were standardised by a group of researchers who developed COSMIN (COnsensus-based Standards for the selection of health Measurement INstruments). The following questionnaires were used for the validation process: the Brazilian version of the *Hip Outcome Score;* the validated Brazilian version of the *Nonarthritic Hip Score* and the *12-Item Short-Form Health Survey.* Reliability was calculated using the psychometric properties of internal consistency and intra-rater test-retest reliability, according to the Cronbach's alpha (score > 0.9) and Intraclass Correlation Coefficient (ICC > 0.9) statistical tests, respectively. Validity was checked using the psychometric properties of construct validity and content validity. Construct validity was calculated by convergent validity ($r > 0.7$) and divergent validity ($r < 0.4$), according to Pearson's correlation coefficient. Content validity was analysed by evidence of questionnaires with a floor effect and/or ceiling effect, which did not occur. The psychometric properties of reliability and validity showed excellent results. Further studies are underway to assess the responsiveness of the Brazilian version of the HOS. The process of validating the Brazilian version of the HOS questionnaire was successfully carried out and has made this quality of life assessment tool valid and reliable for the Brazilian Portuguese language and will thus provide Brazilian doctors and health professionals with an instrument capable of assessing physically active patients with hip diseases without serious degenerative changes.

Keywords: Questionnaires. Hip. Orthopaedics. Hip Outcome Score. Reliability. Validity.

CONTENTS

INTRODUCTION

In 1952, the World Health Organisation (WHO) presented a new concept of health that encompassed not only the absence of disease, but also the presence of physical, mental and social well-being. This event contributed to one of the aims of medicine being to reduce the damage caused by disease and promote better health and quality of life (CICONELLI, 2003).

In the past, patients' clinical changes were only assessed through physical examination and complementary tests, which only provide objective data. But in recent decades, outcomes such as health-related quality of life, measured in functional capacity, pain and personal satisfaction scales, have been emphasised because they make it possible to assess health and the manifestations of the disease in the individual's life from their own subjective perspective. These data corroborate clinical findings and complementary tests and are being used more frequently to inform patient progress and decisions on the most appropriate treatment (CICONELLI, 2003; LOPES et al., 2007).

In recent years, a variety of quality of life assessment instruments, questionnaires and scales have been developed and published that address this type of subjective assessment - since the objective, clinical and complementary examination (laboratory and imaging) is a limited indicator for assessing functional, social and emotional aspects (LOPES et al., 2007). These instruments have scales that assess the patient's perception of their state of health and are influenced by the cultural context in which the individual is inserted. These quality of life instruments measure changes in physical function and in the functional, psychological and social aspects of patients (LOPES et al., 2007; DEL CASTILLO et al., 2012).

There is growing interest in the scientific community in the use of such instruments due to their diverse applications, such as individual or population perception of health status, evaluation of results and effectiveness of treatments, possibility of use in clinical research and economic analyses that focus on treatment costs (LOPES et al., 2007). For this reason, quality of life assessment has been increasingly used in the area of health, especially after its psychometric properties (measurement properties) were proven to be a valid, reproducible parameter. Thus, measuring the impact of the disease on the patient's quality of life is becoming an increasingly important tool (DEL CASTILLO et al., 2012).

CHAPTER 1

THEORETICAL FRAMEWORK

1.1 Quality of life assessment tools

Quality of life assessment instruments can be generic or specific. Generic instruments usually assess the patient in a broader way and are applicable to a wide variety of diseases and populations. They also quantify the patient's perception of their general state of health. However, their disadvantage is that they may not identify more specific aspects of certain diseases (LOPES et al., 2007; DEL CASTILLO et al., 2012).

Specific quality of life assessment instruments are used to evaluate the functional integrity of joints or the development of certain diseases and are widely used in orthopaedic literature. These instruments are capable of verifying changes in the function of a body segment or the evolution of a disease. The greatest advantage of this type of instrument is the ability to detect small changes when they occur, as they have greater specificity and sensitivity in their scales aimed at assessing the joint or disease proposed by the instrument (LOPES et al., 2007; DEL CASTILLO et al., 2012).

1.1.1 Generic quality of life assessment instruments

The 36-Item Short-Form Health Survey (SF-36) was created in 1992 by Ware and Sherbourne. It is easy to administer and consists of 36 items divided into eight subscales: functional capacity, physical aspects, pain, general health, vitality, social aspects, emotional aspects and mental health (WARE; SHERBOURNE, 1992). The SF-36 questionnaire has already been translated and validated in Portuguese (CICONELLI et al., 1999). Despite being a useful quality of life questionnaire that is not specific to joint conditions, the SF-36 has often been used as a reference in orthopaedic literature (ESCOBAR et al., 2002; DEL CASTILLO et al., 2013).

The *12-Item Short-Form Health Survey* (SF-12) is a summarised version of the SF-36:

it was created in 1994 by Ware et al. as a quicker alternative to the SF-36 instrument (WARE et al., 1996). The SF-12 consists of twelve items derived from the SF-36, which assess eight different dimensions of influence on quality of life: physical function, physical aspect, pain, general health, vitality, social function, emotional aspect and mental health; distributed in two sub-scales: physical health and mental health (CAMELIER, 2004; SILVEIRA et al., 2013).

1.1.2 Specific quality of life assessment instruments

Hip-specific questionnaires can be divided into two main groups: to assess patients with severe degenerative joint disease (with osteoarthritis) or without severe degenerative joint disease (without osteoarthritis).

Degenerative joint disease is a chronic multifactorial disease characterised by the degeneration of articular cartilage. Clinically, the patient may present with pain, oedema, morning stiffness, bone crepitus and muscle atrophy. Femoroacetabular impingement (FAI) is considered a clinical precursor to joint degeneration that can lead to osteoarthritis (GANZ et al., 2003; LEUNIG et al., 2005; GANZ et al., 2008). The radiographic characteristics of osteoarthritis are: narrowing of the joint space, presence of osteophytes, sclerosis and resorption of the subchondral bone (COIMBRA et al., 2002).

FAI is characterised by abnormal contact between the femur and the acetabulum. There are other types of impingement, involving the ischium (ischio-femoral impingement) and the anterior inferior iliac spine (subspinal impingement). In FAI, bone impingement usually occurs during flexion, adduction and internal rotation of the hip. There are two basic types of FAI, one characterised by the presence of a gibbosity in the anterolateral region of the femoral head-neck junction (cam deformity) and the other characterised by excess acetabular coverage (pincer deformity), which can be focal or global (Figure 1) (GANZ et al., 2003; LEUNIG et al., 2005; GANZ et al., 2008).

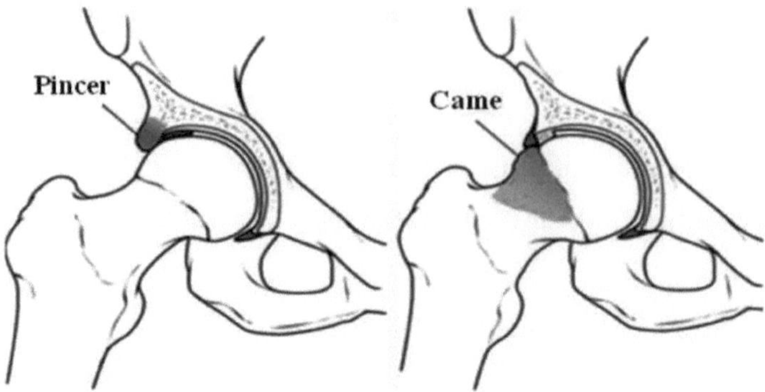

Figure 1 - Femoroacetabular impingement: pincer and cam deformity

Source: ORTHOINFO, 2017, n.p., translated by the author. Reproduced with permission from Orthoinfo.© American Academy of Orthopaedic Surgeons. http://orthoinfo.aaos.org

The cam deformity is characterised radiographically by the presence of an alpha angle of more than 55 degrees in the lateral view of the hip. Focal pincer is related to localised over-coverage, usually by varying degrees of acetabular retroversion, characterised radiographically by the sign of the crossing of the edges, in the anteroposterior view of the hip. Global pincer is a generalised overcoverage of the acetabulum, characterised radiographically by the presence of an acetabular coverage angle (Wiberg's centre-edge angle) above 40 degrees; and it is usually associated with variable degrees of coxa profunda, a condition in which the femoral head is excessively contained by the acetabulum (NEPPLE et al., 2013). Repetitive flexion movements, associated with varying degrees of internal rotation and adduction or abduction, cause lesions in the cartilage and acetabular labrum. The characteristic lesion of pincer FAI is crushing of the superolateral acetabular labrum and degeneration of the postero-inferior chondral surface of the acetabulum (counter-blow lesion). In cam IFA, the characteristic lesion is degeneration at the upper-lateral chondro-labial junction of the acetabulum (GANZ et al., 2003; LEUNIG et al., 2005; GANZ et al., 2008).

The clinical diagnosis of PFMI is usually obtained through the clinical manifestation of pain in the anterior region of the hip or in the gluteal region, related to movements, especially the combination of flexion, adduction and internal rotation, usually reported during physical activity or prolonged sitting (GANZ et al., 2003; GANZ et al., 2008). A clinical manifestation considered pathognomonic of PFI is the "C" sign described by Byrd (2000), in which the patient points to the location of the pain in the hip with their hand in the shape of a "C", in a transverse orientation, which denotes pain of intra-articular origin. Confirmation of the diagnosis of AFI should always be made by finding structural bone abnormalities, which can be done with radiographs of the hip. Other diagnostic imaging methods (computed tomography and nuclear magnetic resonance) help to characterise bone and soft tissue alterations (LEUNIG et al., 2005).

Peritrochanteric Pain Syndrome (PTPS) is a term used to describe chronic or intermittent pain accompanied by tenderness on palpation in the lateral region of the hip. For a long time, the predominant idea was that trochanteric bursitis was the main clinical condition in these cases. The main clinical characteristics related to PTSD found in the literature are local pain exacerbated by forced abduction, hip abduction weakness, pain on flexion, internal or external rotation of the hip and painful palpation of the greater trochanter. Clinical diagnosis is made through physical examinations and diagnostic imaging methods, which seek to identify characteristic local alterations, such as enthesopathy of the gluteus minimus and medius, thickening of the trochanteric bursa and the presence of oedema in the iliotibial tract; and also by excluding degenerative bone pathological processes or tumours, among other conditions (FUJIKI et al., 2008; WILLIAMS et al., 2009).

1.1.2.1 Specific instruments for patients with severe degenerative joint disease

Questionnaires aimed at assessing individuals with severe degenerative joint disease who may be candidates for arthroplasty are: Merle d'Aubigné- Postel Hip Score (MD & Postel), for patients with osteoarthritis of the hip (D'AUBIGNÉ; POSTEL, 1954); Harris Hip Score (HHS), which assesses the results of total hip arthroplasty (HARRIS, 1969); Western Ontario and McMasters Universities Osteoarthritis Index (WOMAC), for patients with osteoarthritis of the hip and knee (BELLAMY et al., 1988a; BELLAMY et al., 1988b); the Oxford Hip Score (OHS), which assesses patients undergoing total hip arthroplasty (DAWSON et al., 1996); the Lequesne Algofunctional Index, aimed at patients with osteoarthritis of the hip and knee (LEQUESNE, 1997); and the Osteoarthritis Knee and Hip Quality of Life (OAKHQOL), for patients with osteoarthritis of the hip and knee (RAT et al., 2005).

Specific questionnaires for individuals with moderate to severe degenerative joint disease of the hip have been developed for patients who are severely limited in their physical and functional capacity. However, these questionnaires show low sensitivity to limitations in high-demand activities because, when applied to a young and physically active population, they usually show the ceiling effect; that is, they achieve the maximum score despite the complaint and performance limitation resulting from the hip problem. According to Safran and Hariri (2010), this can be incorrectly interpreted as a satisfactory result (SAFRAN; HARIRI, 2010).

1.1.2.2 Specific instruments for patients without severe degenerative joint disease

For more physically active individuals without severe degenerative joint disease, questionnaires are used: Nonarthritic Hip Score (NAHS), developed to assess hip function in young patients with hip pain (CHRISTENSEN et al., 2003); Hip Disability and Osteoarthritis Outcome Score (HOOS), suitable for assessing patients with or without hip osteoarthritis (KLÀSSBO et al., 2003, NILSDOTTER et al., 2003); *Hip Outcome Score* (HOS), which assesses the results of therapeutic interventions in physically active individuals with acetabular labrum lesions (MARTIN, 2005); *Hip and Groin Outcome Score* (HAGOS), for young patients with hip pain (THORBORG et al., 2011); the *International Hip Outcome Tool* (iHOT 12/33), for patients with hip disorders (MOHTADI et al., 2012); and the *Hip Sports Activity Scale* (HSAS), which is a scale that assesses the level of sports activity in patients with AFI (NAAL et al., 2013).

Hip pain caused by acetabular labrum injury in young, physically active patients has generated growing interest among orthopaedic surgeons, physiotherapists and other health professionals due to the recognised importance of acetabular labrum injury as one of the factors involved in the origin of degenerative joint disease of the hip (LEUNIG et al., 2005).

The *Nonarthritic Hip Score* (NAHS) and *Hip Outcome Score* (HOS) questionnaires are widely used to assess these patients (DEL CASTILLO et al., 2013; OLIVEIRA et al., 2014).

The *Nonarthritic Hip Score* (NAHS) questionnaire was developed by Christensen et al. in 2003 in the United States of America (USA) to assess hip function in young, physically active patients with hip pain. The NAHS questionnaire consists of 20 questions and has four domains: ten questions that address pain and function, four questions about mechanical symptoms and six questions about the level of physical activity (CHRISTENSEN et al., 2003).

The Hip Outcome Score (HOS) questionnaire was developed by Martin in 2005 in the USA to assess physically active and/or young patients with acetabular labrum lesions (MARTIN, 2005). This questionnaire has been validated to measure function in individuals undergoing hip arthroscopy and with acetabular labrum damage (MARTIN et al., 2006; MARTIN; PHILIPPON, 2007). The HOS is made up of 28 items divided into two sub-scales, 19 items on activities of daily living (ADL) and nine items exclusively on sporting activities (Sport) (MARTIN, 2005). A 2010 systematic review of various hip-specific questionnaires concluded that the HOS is the most recommended questionnaire for assessing young patients undergoing hip arthroscopy (THORBORG et al., 2010).

1.2 Translation and cultural adaptation of quality of life assessment instruments

Most quality of life and orthopaedic assessment instruments were created in English (HARRIS, 1969; DAWSON et al., 1996; CHRISTENSEN et al., 2003; MARTIN, 2005). For these instruments to be used in a population with a different language and culture to the country in which they were developed, it is necessary to follow a number of stages for their translation, cultural adaptation to the language and, finally, their validation, from which the new instrument will be assessed as to whether it maintains the psychometric properties of the original instrument (GUILLEMIN et al., 1993; BEATON et al., 2000; SCHOLTES et al., 2011).

A set of standardised instructions for the translation and cultural adaptation of quality of life assessment instruments includes five stages: translation, synthesis, back translation, committee review and pre-testing. These criteria were described by Guillemin et al. (1993) and revised by Beaton et al. (2000). After these translation and cultural adaptation stages, the assessment instrument must have its psychometric properties (measurement properties) tested, i.e. validated (MOKKINK et al., 2006; SCHOLTES et al., 2011; MOKKINK et al., 2016).

1.3 Validation of quality of life assessment instruments

Psychometric properties verify that the new version of the instrument has maintained the characteristics of the original instrument. The domains commonly studied for the validation process are reliability, validity and responsiveness (MOKKINK et al., 2006; SCHOLTES et al., 2011).

These domains were standardised by a group of researchers who developed the COnsensus-based Standards for the selection of health Measurement Instruments (COSMIN), which is a consensus-based guideline for the selection of quality of life and health assessment instruments and also for assessing the methodological quality of studies using psychometric properties (MOKKINK et al., 2006; MOKKINK et al., 2010a; MOKKINK et al., 2016). In addition, these researchers have defined the terminologies and definitions of these psychometric properties. These standardised criteria were established through the international and multidisciplinary Delphi study, in which several experts from various countries took part (MOKKINK et al., 2006; MOKKINK et al., 2010a; MOKKINK et al., 2010b; SCHOLTES et al., 2011).

According to COSMIN, the reliability domain contains the psychometric properties of internal consistency, reliability and measurement error; while the validity domain consists of analysing construct validity, content validity and criterion validity (MOKKINK et al., 2010a; MOKKINK et al., 2010b; SCHOLTES et al., 2011; MOKKINK et al., 2016).

1.3.1 Reliability

The reliability domain contains three psychometric properties: internal consistency, reliability (test-retest, inter-rater and intra-rater) and measurement error. This domain refers to the degree to which the instrument is free of measurement errors and, at the same time, also assesses the questionnaire's ability to present similar results when the same patients are assessed at different times, but without any changes in their state of health (MOKKINK et al., 2006; MOKKINK et al., 2010b; SCHOLTES et al., 2011; MOKKINK et al., 2016).

These psychometric properties can be assessed in the following ways:

a. Using different sets of items from the same measuring instrument (internal consistency);
b. Over time (test-retest);
c. By different assessors on the same occasion (inter-assessor);
d. By the same individual (assessors or patients) on different occasions (intra-assessor).

Each of these properties estimates reliability in a different way (MOKKINK et al., 2006; MOKKINK et al., 2010b; SCHOLTES et al., 2011; MOKKINK et al., 2016).

1.1.1.1 Internal consistency

Internal consistency assesses the ability of a group of questions to measure a similar concept. It is measured by estimating the degree of interrelationship between the items (questions). In other words, if the items on a scale are grouped together in the same total score, it must be proven that these items are considerably correlated. Internal consistency establishes this correlation between the items in a quality of life assessment instrument. The estimate of

Internal consistency differs from other reliability estimates because there is no repeated administration of the measuring instrument (MOKKINK et al., 2010b; SCHOLTES et al., 2011; MOKKINK et al., 2016).

1.1.1.2 Reliability

It is the proportion of the total variance in measurements due to true differences between patients. Reliability can be assessed through: test-retest reliability, inter-rater reliability and intra-rater reliability (MOKKINK et al., 2010b; SCHOLTES et al., 2011; MOKKINK et al., 2016).

1.1.1.2.1 Test-retest reliability

Test-retest reliability assesses reliability at different points in time. It is estimated by administering a measuring instrument, such as a questionnaire, on two different occasions to the same group of patients. This psychometric property assesses the ability of an assessment instrument to provide similar results when the same patients are assessed at different times, but without any changes in their state of health (MOKKINK et al., 2010b; SCHOLTES et al., 2011; MOKKINK et al., 2016).

Test-retest reliability is based on the hypothesis that no real change has occurred between what is measured. Therefore, the ideal time interval between measurements should be long enough so that the last score is not influenced by memorising the first, because if the interval is too short, it could overestimate reliability. However, this time interval should also not be too long, so that the subject has actually changed their state of health in this time interval, underestimating reliability (MOKKINK et al., 2010b; SCHOLTES et al., 2011; MOKKINK et al., 2016).

1.1.1.2.2 Inter-rater reliability

Inter-rater reliability assesses the reliability between different raters at the same time. It assesses whether there is consensus in the scores of two evaluators when the same measuring instrument is used. This psychometric property can be estimated by having both evaluators administer the same instrument, on the same patient, or at the same time in a group of patients (SCHOLTES et al., 2011 MOKKINK et al., 2016).

1.1.1.2.3 Intra-rater reliability

Intra-rater reliability assesses reliability through measurements obtained by the same people at different times. It is measured when an evaluator applies the same instrument on two different occasions to the same patient. Or when a patient answers the same questionnaire alone, for example, at two different times. Both intra- and inter-rater reliability are based on good rater training and standardisation (SCHOLTES et al., 2011; MOKKINK et al., 2016).

1.1.1.3 Measurement error

Measurement error is made up of systematic and random errors in patients' test-retest scores, which are not attributed to real changes in the construct being measured. Measurement error refers to the absolute amount of measurement error, and variation between individuals does not affect measurement error. The statistic used to express measurement error is the Standard Error of Measurement (SEM). The Minimum Clinical Difference (MCD) is directly related to the MSE. Due to the absolute nature of the measurement error, both are measured on the same scale with the instrument itself. EPM represents the standard deviation of repeated measurements of an individual. The DCM represents the minimum change that must be exceeded to guarantee real change. Knowledge of the amount of measurement error contributes to clinical relevance when the results of instruments are used for evaluation purposes, such as assessing the effect of surgery or other treatments, and can be used to decide whether a clinically relevant change has occurred in the patient (SCHOLTES et al., 2011; MOKKINK et al., 2016).

Agreement is the graphical representation of measurement errors between the test and retest using the Bland-Altman (ALTMAN; BLAND, 1983; BLAND; ALTMAN, 1986) and agreement-survival (LUIZ et al., 2003) graphs, which quantify agreement by means of limits of agreement based on the mean test-retest scores and the differences between the two assessments. These statistical limits are calculated using the mean and standard deviation of the differences between the two assessments.

1.3.2 Expiry date

The validity domain refers to the degree to which the instrument measures the concept it intends to measure (MOKKINK et al., 2010b). Validity contains three psychometric properties: construct validity, content validity and criterion validity (SCHOLTES et al., 2011; MOKKINK et al., 2016).

1.3.2.1 Validity of construction

Construct validity represents the degree to which an instrument's scores are consistent with the hypotheses, based on the assumption that the validated instrument measures the proposed construct (MOKKINK et al., 2010b). Hypotheses are established about expected internal relationships, relationships with the results of other instruments, or expected differences in results between the relevant groups. There is no consensus on the number of hypotheses that should be tested or confirmed in order to assert adequate construct validity. Some authors suggest that 75 per cent of the hypotheses should be confirmed (SCHOLTES et al., 2011; MOKKINK et al., 2016).

1.3.2.2 Content validity

Content validity represents the degree to which the content of a measuring instrument can be considered an adequate reflection of the construct being measured (MOKKINK et al., 2010b). Content validity also contains face validity, which defines the degree to which the items in a measuring instrument do, in fact, appear to be an adequate reflection of the construct being measured. However, there are no standards for what is acceptable content validity, because this requires subjective judgement (SCHOLTES et al., 2011; MOKKINK et al., 2016). However, one way of assessing content validity can be through the evidence of questionnaires with a score of zero or a maximum score of 100, i.e. the floor effect and the ceiling effect (EVERITT; SKRONDAL, 2010).

1.3.2.3 Validity of criteria

According to the researchers who developed COSMIN, criterion validity is determined by the degree to which the scores of an instrument show themselves to be an adequate reflection of an instrument classified as a "gold standard". Thus, criterion validity can only be assessed when the criterion used is reasonably considered a "gold standard". Paradoxically, however, these same researchers have reached a consensus that there is no health assessment instrument classified as a "gold standard" (MOKKJNK et al., 2010b; SCHOLTES et al., 2011).

1.3.3 Responsiveness

It is the ability of a measuring instrument to detect changes over time in the construct being measured. It is estimated by repeatedly administering the instrument on two different occasions over a long period of time to the same group of patients. However, there is no consensus on the best way to assess this domain (SCHOLTES et al., 2011; MOKKINK et al., 2016).

CHAPTER 2

RELEVANCE OF THE STUDY

The Hip Outcome Score (HOS) is an instrument capable of assessing young and/or physically active patients with hip disease without serious degenerative changes (MARTIN, 2005), a condition that other hip assessment instruments are not able to fulfil with the same specificity (CHRISTENSEN et al., 2003; KLÀSSBO et al., 2003; MOHTADI et al., 2012; NAAL et al., 2013). The NAHS questionnaire, although it has questions about the level of physical activity, does not have a sports activities subscale like the HOS, which calculates this score separately. A 2010 systematic review of various hip-specific questionnaires concluded that the HOS questionnaire is the most recommended for assessing young patients undergoing hip arthroscopy (THORBORG et al., 2010).

The hip research group at the Pedro Ernesto University Hospital of the State University of Rio de Janeiro (HUPE/UERJ) has already carried out the translation and cultural adaptation stages of the HOS questionnaire, generating the Brazilian version of the HOS (HOS-Brasil) (OLIVEIRA et al., 2014). However, it has not yet been validated, i.e. it remains to be seen whether this version has maintained the psychometric properties of the original instrument.

As there is a great need to assess this specific group of patients (OLIVEIRA et al., 2014), the validation of the Hip Outcome Score for the Brazilian Portuguese language is extremely important. The use of this validated questionnaire will provide doctors and health professionals in Brazil with a more specific hip assessment tool for young and/or physically active patients with hip diseases without serious degenerative changes.

CHAPTER 3

OBJECTIVES

3.1 General objective

The aim of this study is to validate the Brazilian version of the Hip Outcome Score (HOS-Brazil) questionnaire, which assesses the hip without serious degenerative changes, in a group of physically active patients with a medical diagnosis of femoroacetabular impingement or peritrochanteric pain syndrome.

3.2 Specific objectives

I. Measuring the psychometric properties of Reliability:
   i. Internal consistency
   ii. Reliability (intra-rater test-retest)
   iii. Measurement error

II. Measuring the psychometric properties of Validity:
   i. Content validity
   ii. Validity of construction

CHAPTER 4

METHODS

4.1 Study design

This master's thesis consisted of an epidemiological, observational, cross-sectional, descriptive, non-controlled study.

4.2 Ethics Committee

This study was previously approved by the Research Ethics Committee of the Pedro Ernesto University Hospital of the State University of Rio de Janeiro, under CEP/HUPE number 2674 (Appendices A and B). The patients were briefed on the objectives of the study and the methodology used before signing the Informed Consent Form (ICF) (Appendix A). Authorisation was obtained from the author of the Hip Outcome Score questionnaire for its translation into Brazilian Portuguese, adaptation to Brazilian culture and validation.

4.3 Patient selection

A total of 70 physically active patients of both genders with complaints of hip pain and a medical diagnosis of femoroacetabular impingement or peritrochanteric pain syndrome were selected.

Literate patients, regardless of gender and ethnicity, complaining of hip pain and with a medical diagnosis of femoroacetabular impingement, confirmed by radiographic or tomographic examinations, or patients with a medical diagnosis of peritrochanteric pain syndrome, confirmed by nuclear magnetic resonance imaging, were included.

Patients were excluded: those with visual or cognitive disorders that prevented them from reading and interpreting the questionnaires; those with hip arthrosis, characterised by a minimum joint space of less than 1.5 mm and severe limitation of the hip's range of movement (CROFT et al., 1990); those who did not fully answer the questionnaires on the first day and after an interval of 48 hours after the first application.

The patients were selected consecutively at the hip outpatient clinic of the Instituto Ortopédico da Tijuca, a private healthcare institution in the city of Rio de Janeiro (RJ). Data was collected between December 2014 and June 2016. The patients selected for the study were briefed on the objectives of the study and answered the research protocol in a private, air-conditioned room.

4.4 Research protocol

The research protocol consisted of signing the Informed Consent Form (ICF) (Appendix A); filling in the identification and clinical assessment form with the clinical characteristics of each patient (Appendix B); and applying the following three quality of life assessment instruments: Brazilian and validated version of the 12-Item Short-Form Health Survey (SF-12) (Appendix C), Brazilian and validated version of the Nonarthritic Hip Score (NAHS) (Appendix D), Brazilian version of the Hip Outcome Score (HOS-Brasil) (Appendix E).

All the patients were instructed to initially answer all three questionnaires (1st application or test) and, after a 48-hour interval, to answer only the Brazilian version of the HOS-Brazil questionnaire (2nd application or retest) via e-mail.

4.4.1 Validated Brazilian version of the *12-Item Short-Form Health Survey* (SF-12)

The SF-12 consists of 12 items and assesses eight different dimensions of influence on quality of life: physical function, physical aspect, pain, general health, vitality, social function, emotional aspect and mental health. This questionnaire considers the individual's perception of aspects of their health in the four weeks prior to its application (SILVEIRA et al., 2013).

Using a proprietary algorithm, two sub-scales can be measured: physical *(Physical Component Summary,* or PCS) and mental *(Mental Component Summary,* or MCS). In both, the score ranges from zero to 100, with higher scores being associated with better levels of quality of life. The questions that assess physical function, physical aspect, pain and general health have higher correlations with the physical subscale, while vitality, social function, emotional aspect and mental health are more correlated with the mental subscale (WARE et al., 1995; GANDEK et al., 1998; SILVEIRA et al., 2013).

The Brazilian Portuguese version of the SF-12 was validated in two populations. In 2004, for a population with chronic obstructive pulmonary disease (CAMELIER, 2004); and, in 2013, for a sample of the population of the city of Montes Claros (MG) through an epidemiological survey of oral health (SILVEIRA et al., 2013).

4.4.2 Brazilian and validated version of the *Nonarthritic Hip Score* (NAHS)

The NAHS is a simple, self-administered questionnaire for assessing hip function in young and/or physically active patients. The questionnaire consists of 20 questions, five of which refer to pain, four to mechanical symptoms, five to function and six to level of physical activity. Each of these 20 questions has five options

answer. Each response corresponds to a specific value and these values are added together at the end of the assessment and multiplied by 1.25 - resulting in the final score. A maximum value of 100 indicates that the patient has normal hip function (DEL CASTILLO et al., 2013).

The NAHS questionnaire, originally developed in English in the USA, was translated into Brazilian Portuguese, adapted for Brazilian culture and validated for Brazil by Del Castillo et al. (2013).

4.4.3 <u>Brazilian version of the *Hip Outcome Score* (HOS-Brazil)</u>

The HOS is a self-administered questionnaire with 28 items (questions) divided into two subscales, one for Activities of Daily Living (ADL), with 19 items, and the other for Sport, with nine items (MARTIN, 2005; OLIVEIRA et al., 2014). Each subscale's final score can vary between 0 and 100, with higher scores representing better hip function. Each subscale has its score calculated separately (MARTIN et al., 2006).

Each of the 28 items has the same five answer options and each answer corresponds to a specific score, which generates a sum at the end of the assessment. The answer to each of the 19 items in the ADL subscale is scored between 4 and 0, with 4 indicating "no difficulty" and 0 indicating "cannot perform". The scores for each of the items are added together to obtain the total score for the items. The total score of the items answered by the patient is multiplied by 4 to obtain the highest potential score. If the patient answers all 19 items, the highest potential score is 76. This total score obtained is divided by the maximum potential score - in this case, for the ADL subscale, it will be 76. This value obtained is then multiplied by 100 to calculate a percentage. The nine items of the Sport subscale are calculated in a similar way, with the highest potential score being 36. The highest final score represents a higher level of physical function for both the ADL and Sport subscales (MARTIN et al., 2006).

In addition, the HOS presents two questions about how the patient would quantify, on a scale of 0 to 100, their functional level in ADL and Sport; and also a qualitative question about their current functional level (normal, almost normal, abnormal, very abnormal). However, these three questions are not included in the final HOS score (SEIJAS et al., 2014).

The original HOS was developed in English in the USA (MARTIN, 2005) (Appendix F). The Brazilian version of the HOS was translated and culturally adapted by OLIVEIRA et al. (2014).

4.5 Statistical analysis

A descriptive statistical analysis was used to characterise the study population. The psychometric properties of reliability and validity needed to validate the Brazilian version of the HOS questionnaire were statistically analysed using GraphPad Prism software, version 7.00 for Windows (GraphPad Software, La Jolla, California, USA).

4.5.1 Reliability

The reliability domain of the Brazilian version of the HOS was assessed using three properties: internal consistency, intra-rater test-retest reliability and measurement error (MOKKINK et al., 2010b; SCHOLTES et al., 2011; MOKKINK et al., 2016).

To calculate internal consistency, Cronbach's alpha was used to check the correlations between the variability of the answers in the questionnaire, assessing the set of questions in each sub-scale separately (CRONBACH, 1951; HAIR et al., 2009). In addition, Cronbach's alpha was recalculated after removing each question or item in isolation to check whether there was a change in the results and whether the question was really necessary.

Intra-rater test-retest reliability was calculated on the 70 selected patients who initially answered the full study protocol and, after a 48-hour interval, answered only the Brazilian version of the HOS (2ª application or retest) by e-mail. During this time interval, no new medication, therapy or procedure was introduced that could rapidly modify the patient's clinical condition.

To assess intra-rater test-retest reliability, the Intraclass Correlation Coefficient (ICC) was used, which is an estimate of the fraction of the total variability of the measurements due to variations between individuals. To do this, the questionnaire had to be administered at two different times to the same patient. These two moments were evaluated using the ICC, which checked whether they reproduced the same effects at two moments. An ICC between 0.4 and 0.75 is considered satisfactory, with an ICC > 0.75 being excellent (BARTKO, 1966).

The paired Student's t-test was used to compare and evaluate the difference between the first and second application of the HOS. The paired Student's t-test calculates the difference between each pair of measurements before (1st application or test) and after (2nd application or retest), determines the average of these changes and reports whether this average of the differences is statistically significant ($p < 0.05$) (VIEIRA, 2010).

Measurement error was assessed by calculating the Standard Error of Measurement (SEM) and the Minimum Clinical Difference (MCD). The MSE was calculated by multiplying the square root of 1 minus the ICC by the standard deviation of the scores from the first application of the Brazilian version of the HOS. The MCD was calculated by multiplying the MPE by 1.96, equivalent to the z score relative to the 95% confidence interval (CI), and the square root of 2 (BARTLETT; FROST, 2008; SCHOLTES et al., 2011).

Concordance was established using the Bland-Altman (ALTMAN; BLAND, 1983; BLAND; ALTMAN, 1986) and concordance-survival (LUIZ et al., 2003) graphs. A linear regression curve of the Bland-Altman graph was calculated to assess the presence of a proportional bias (ALTMAN; BLAND, 1983;
BLAND; ALTMAN, 1986). The independent variable (x-axis) used to carry out the linear regression was the average of the two assessments and the dependent variable (y-axis) was the difference between the two assessments. The null hypothesis was that the slope of the regression line would not differ from zero. Proportional bias refers to the scenario in which the difference between two measurements is not constant over the entire possible range of scores, as indicated by the p-value of the angular coefficient of the regression curve being statistically significant ($p < 0.05$). If the difference in scores between the two measurement occasions is constant, regardless of the magnitude of the score, then it is described as a fixed bias (ALTMAN; BLAND, 1983; BLAND; ALTMAN, 1986).

4.5.2 Expiry date

The domain validity of the Brazilian version of the HOS was assessed using the psychometric properties of construct validity and content validity (MOKKINK et al., 2010b; SCHOLTES et al., 2011; MOKKINK et al., 2016).

To assess construct validity, the Brazilian version of the HOS (OLIVEIRA et al., 2014) was completed by the patients along with the Brazilian and validated versions of the questionnaires: NAHS (DEL CASTILLO et al., 2013) and SF- 12 (SILVEIRA et al., 2013). The aim of construct validity was to verify the convergent and divergent construct validities present in the Brazilian version of the HOS questionnaire, when compared to the other two questionnaires applied.

For convergent construct validity, the correlations of the scores of the HOS (ADL and Sport subscale), NAHS (total score) and SF-12 (Physical subscale) questionnaires were assessed. For divergent construct validity, the correlations between the scores on the HOS questionnaires (ADL and Sport subscales) and the SF-12 questionnaire (Mental subscale) were assessed. The convergent and divergent construct validities were assessed under the hypotheses that the SF-12 Physical subscale score and the NAHS total score should have a moderate to high correlation with the HOS ADL and Sport subscales. In addition, it is expected to find a higher correlation between the HOS and the NAHS because they are specific instruments for assessing the hip. On the other hand, we should find a low correlation between the scores on the ADL and Sports subscales of the HOS and the score on the Mental subscale of the SF-12.

To assess convergent construct validity, it is necessary to find a strong and significant correlation between the compared variables, because it is expected that the two, despite being part of different questionnaires, will have the same direction. With regard to divergent construct validity, the exact opposite is expected: a weak and non-significant correlation must be found. To assess both convergent and divergent construct validity, Pearson's correlation coefficient was used, which generates an indicator that can vary from -1 (perfect negative correlation) to +1 (perfect positive correlation), where a value of zero indicates no correlation between the variables studied (VIEIRA, 2010).

The content validity of the Brazilian version of the HOS was assessed by the evidence of questionnaires with the floor effect and ceiling effect. The ceiling effect can be observed when there are evaluations that reach the maximum possible score of the questionnaire, 100 (one hundred). The floor effect occurs when there are evaluations with the minimum possible score, 0 (zero) (EVERITT; SKRONDAL, 2010).

CHAPTER 5

RESULTS

5.1 Patient characteristics

Seventy physically active patients with complaints of hip pain were selected. Table 1 shows the profile of these patients. All were literate and answered the questionnaires themselves. They were selected consecutively at the hip outpatient clinic of the Tijuca Orthopaedic Institute in the city of Rio de Janeiro (RJ). Appendix C shows the individual clinical characteristics of the 70 patients selected.

Table 1 - Patient profile

Gender	Female	46 (65,7%)
	Male	24 (34,3%)
Age	Mean (SD)	42,9 (12,9)
Medical Diagnosis	Femoroacetabular impingement	26 (37,1%)
	Peritrochanteric pain syndrome	44 (62,9%)

Legend: standard deviation (SD).
Source: The author, 2017.

5.2 Results of the questionnaires

Table 2 shows the mean, standard deviation (SD), minimum and maximum scores for the NAHS, SF-12 and HOS questionnaires.

Table 2 - Questionnaire scores applied to the 70 patients

Questionnaires	**Average**	**DP**	**Min. score**	**Max. score**
NAHS - Total score	62,0	21,8	12,5	96,2
SF-12 - Mental subscale	52,2	9,5	15,8	65,1
SF-12 - Physical subscale	42,9	12,5	20,8	60,9
1st HOS application - ADL subscale	71,1	18,1	25,0	97,4
1st HOS application - Sport subscale	55,1	23,7	2,8	97,2
2nd HOS application - ADL subscale	71,0	17,8	26,3	98,6
2nd HOS application - Sport subscale	55,0	23,3	5,5	97,2

Legend: standard deviation (SD); minimum (Min.); maximum (Max.); Hip Outcome Score (HOS); Activities of Daily Living (ADL); Nonarthritic Hip Score (NAHS); 12-Item Short-Form Health Survey (SF-12).
Source: The author, 2017.

The scores on the three questionnaires ranged from two to 99 points, with higher scores being associated with better quality of life (SF - 12) and better hip function (NAHS and HOS).

5.3 Psychometric properties

5.3.1 Reliability

5.3.1.1 Internal consistency

Table 3 shows the results of the internal consistency analysis for the 1st (test) application of the HOS. According to Hair et al. (2009), the minimum recommended value for Cronbach's alpha is 0.7. If the result for Cronbach's alpha varies between 0.8 and 0.9, it is considered to be moderate to high reliability; and above 0.9 it is considered to be high reliability.

Table 3 - Internal consistency by Cronbach's alpha

Questionnaire	Sub-scale	Cronbach's alpha
1ª HOS application	AVD	0,95
	Sport	0,92

Legend: Hip Outcome Score (HOS); Activities of Daily Living (ADL).
Source: The author, 2017.

Table 4 shows that the removal of any single question or item did not significantly alter the results found by Cronbach's alpha in each of the sub-scales analysed (Table 4).

Table 4 - Internal consistency by Cronbach's alpha when removing each question

HOS issues	DLA subscale	Sport subscale
1	0,95	0,91
2	0,94	0,90
3	0,94	0,92
4	0,94	0,91

5	0,95	0,91
6	0,94	0,92
7	0,94	0,92
8	0,94	0,92
9	0,94	0,92
10	0,94	-
11	0,95	-
12	0,95	-
13	0,95	-
14	0,95	-
15	0,95	-
16	0,95	-
17	0,94	-
18	0,94	-
19	0,94	-

Legend: Hip Outcome Score (HOS); Activities of Daily Living (ADL). Source: The author, 2017.

5.3.1.2 Intra-rater test-retest reliability

The ICC value obtained in the Brazilian version of the HOS was 0.99 for the two subscales, and the confidence interval (95% CI) varied between 0.986-0.995 for the ADL subscale and between 0.990-0.996 for the Sport subscale (Table 5). An ICC between 0.4 and 0.75 is considered satisfactory, with an ICC > 0.75 being excellent.

Table 5 - Intra-assessor test-retest reliability

Comparison	**HOS subscales**	**JRC**	**95%IC INF**	**95%IC SUP**
1ª application - 2ª application from HOS	AVD	0,992	0,986	0,995
	Sport	0,994	0,990	0,996

Legend: Hip Outcome Score (HOS); Intraclass Correlation Coefficient (ICC); Activities of Daily Living (ADL); Confidence Interval (CI); lower (INF); upper (SUP).
Source: The author, 2017.

5.3.1.3 Measurement error and agreement

The paired Student's t-test showed no statistically significant differences between the mean test-retest values of the HOS ADL subscale ($p = 0.84$) and the HOS Sport subscale ($p = 0.82$). The limits of agreement and the confidence interval were analysed. The Bland-

Altman plot indicated a mean error of difference between the scores obtained in the two HOS assessments of -0.1 for the two HOS subscales (95% limit of agreement = -4.5 to 4.5 for the ADL subscale and -5.3 to 5.2 for the Sport subscale of the HOS). The two dotted lines represent the upper and lower limits of agreement. The p-value of the angular coefficient of the regression curve revealed that the slope of the curve did not deviate significantly from zero (P = 0.26 in the ADL subscale and P = 0.14 in the Sport subscale of the HOS) (Figures 2 and 3).

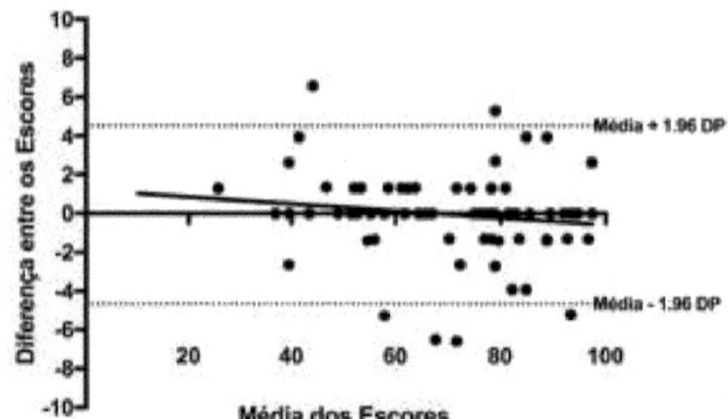

Figure 2 - Bland-Altman graph showing the difference between the two assessments of the HOS ADL subscale

Legend: Hip Outcome Score (HOS); Activities of Daily Living (ADL). Source: The author, 2017.

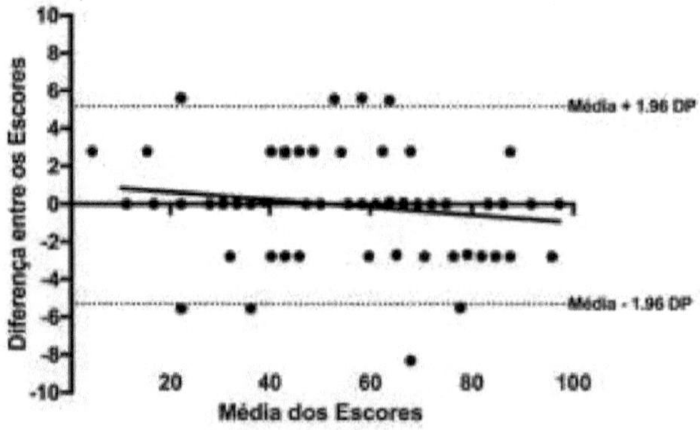

Figure 3 - Bland-Altman graph showing the difference between the two assessments of the Sport subscale of the HOS

Caption: Hip Outcome Score (HOS). Source: The author, 2017.

The EPM found for the ADL subscale was 1.7 points; for the Sport subscale it was 1.9 points. The DCM calculated was 4.6 points on the ADL subscale and 5.3 points on the Sports subscale of the Brazilian version of the HOS.

The concordance-survival graphs are shown in Figures 4 and 5 and reveal two aspects: a 7-point difference in the ADL subscale (Figure 4) and a 6-point difference in the Sports subscale (Figure 5) - which represent a 95 per cent concordance of the test-retest scores of the Brazilian version of the HOS.

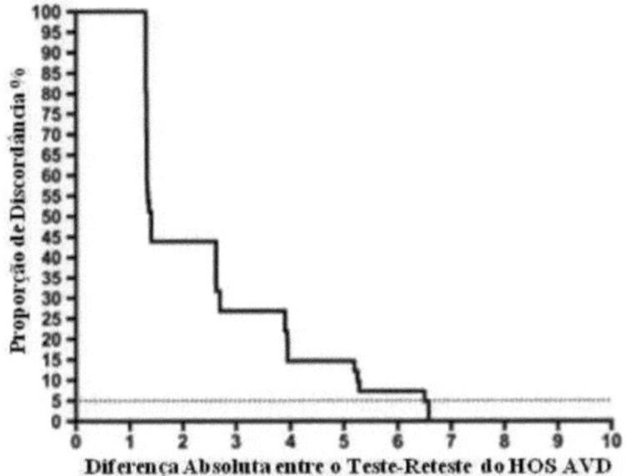

Figure 4 - Agreement-survival graph for the HOS ADL subscale
Legend: Hip Outcome Score (HOS); Activities of Daily Living (ADL).
Source: The author, 2017.

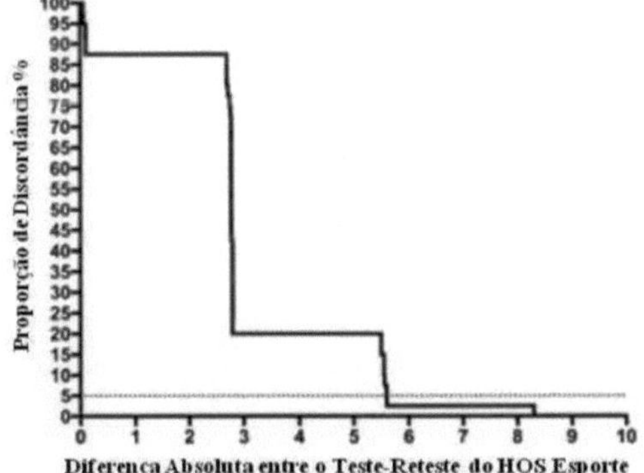

Figure 5 - Agreement-survival graph for the Sport subscale of the HOS
Caption: Hip Outcome Score (HOS). Source: The author, 2017.

5.3.2 Expiry date

5.3.2.1 Validity of construction

Convergent construct validity was calculated using Pearson's correlation coefficient (r) by correlating the scores of the HOS ADL and Sport subscales (1ª application or test) with the total score generated by the NAHS and the SF-12 Physical subscale score. The values of the coefficients found in the correlations were greater than 0.7; with the exception of the correlation of the HOS Sport subscale with the SF-12 Physical subscale, which was 0.685 - indicating high and moderate correlations, respectively (Table 6).

Table 6 - Pearson's correlation coefficient for convergent construct validity

Questionnaires (sub-scale)	Pearson (r)
HOS (ADL subscale) x NAHS (total score)	0,874
HOS (ADL subscale) x SF-12 (Physical subscale)	0,744
HOS (Sport subscale) x NAHS (total score)	0,789
HOS (Sport subscale) x SF-12 (Physical subscale)	0,685

Key: Hip Outcome Score (HOS); Activities of Daily Living (ADL); Nonarthritic Hip Score (NAHS); 12-Item Short-Form Health Survey (SF-12).
Source: The author, 2017.

Next, the divergent construct validity between the HOS and SF-12 questionnaires was checked, as shown in Table 7. Pearson's correlation coefficient was calculated to check for the presence of a correlation between the HOS ADL and Sports subscale scores and the SF-12 Mental subscale score. The results found were lower than 0.4 - indicating low correlations (Table 7).

Table 7 - Pearson's correlation coefficient for divergent construct validity

Questionnaires (sub-scale)	Pearson (r)
HOS (ADL subscale) x SF-12 (Mental subscale)	0,346
HOS (Sports subscale) x SF-12 (Mental subscale)	0,344

Legend: Hip Outcome Score (HOS); Activities of Daily Living (ADL); 12-Item Short-Form Health Survey (SF-12).
Source: The author, 2017.

5.3.2.2 Content validity

The Brazilian version of the HOS had good content validity and there were no questionnaires with a score of zero and/or a maximum score of 100, i.e. there was no floor effect and/or ceiling effect (Figures 6 and 7).

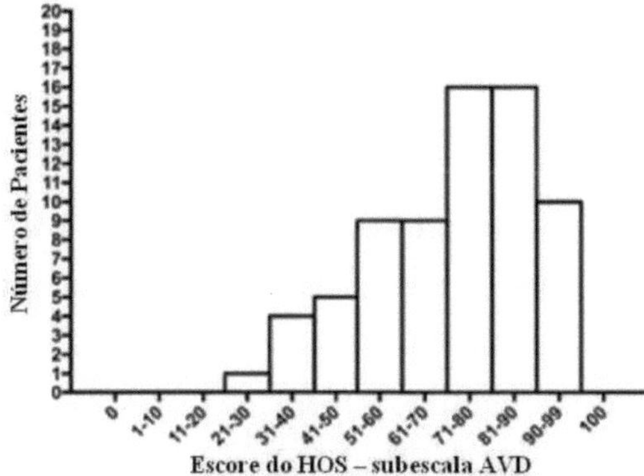

Figure 6 - Distribution of HOS ADL subscale scores in the first application

Legend: Hip Outcome Score (HOS); Activities of Daily Living (ADL).
Source: The author, 2017.

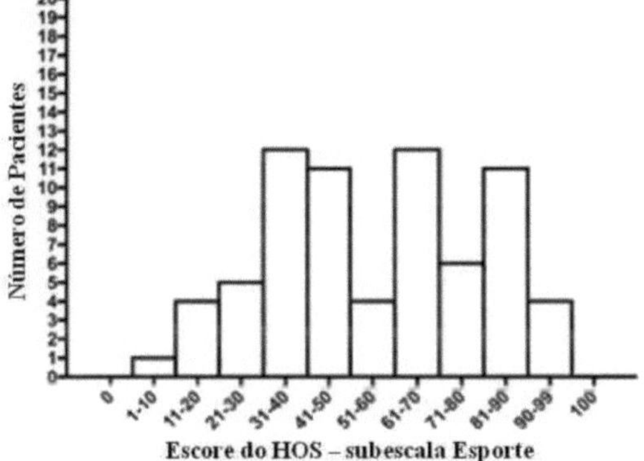

Figure 7 - Distribution of HOS Sport subscale scores in the first application

Caption: Hip Outcome Score (HOS). Source: The author, 2017.

CHAPTER 6

DISCUSSION

The HOS questionnaire is a hip-specific quality of life assessment tool that was originally developed in English (MARTIN, 2005). It has been translated and culturally adapted into German (NAAL et al., 2011), Korean (LEE et al., 2014), Spanish (SEIJAS et al., 2014) and Brazilian Portuguese (OLIVEIRA et al., 2014). The German, Korean and Spanish versions have already been validated in their countries.

In this validation study of the Brazilian version of the HOS questionnaire (HOS-Brazil), a group of physically active patients with a medical diagnosis of femoroacetabular impingement or peritrochanteric pain syndrome was selected. In the validation study of the German version of the HOS, the patients had undergone surgical treatment for femoroacetabular impingement (NAAL et al., 2011). In the validation of the Spanish version, the patients had symptomatic hip disease and underwent surgical treatment for hip arthroscopy (SEIJAS et al., 2014). And in the validation of the Korean version, the patients also underwent hip arthroscopy, but the assessments were carried out before the surgical treatment (LEE et al., 2014).

To validate the Brazilian version of the HOS questionnaire, 70 patients were assessed, with an average age of 42.9 years. For the validation of the German version, 85 patients were assessed, with a mean age of 33.4 years (NAAL et al., 2011); for the Spanish version, there were 100 patients, with a mean age of 45.0 years (SEIJAS et al., 2014); for the Korean version, 60 patients, with a mean age of 38.4 years (LEE et al., 2014). It was therefore found that the mean age of the patients in the study of the Brazilian version of the HOS was similar to the validation studies of the German, Spanish and Korean versions. The sample size of the present study was larger than that assessed by the Korean version study; however, it was smaller than the sample of the German and Spanish version studies.

In the validation of the Brazilian version of the HOS, there was a prevalence of females (65.7%), similar to the result found in the validation of the original HOS in English (54.1%) (MARTIN et al., 2006); and in the evaluation of its reliability and responsiveness (67%)

(MARTIN; PHILIPPON, 2008). However, these findings differ from the validation studies of the German (NAAL et al., 2011), Spanish (SEIJAS et al., 2014) and Korean (LEE et al., 2014) versions, whose prevalence was male, with 57.6%, 64% and 56.7%, respectively.

In this study, the internal consistency of the Brazilian version of the HOS was assessed separately in the two subscales, ADL and Sport, by Cronbach's alpha and showed high reliability with scores above 0.9 for both subscales (0.95 for ADL and 0.92 for Sport). According to Hair et al. (2009), the minimum recommended value for Cronbach's alpha is 0.7; between 0.8 and 0.9 is considered moderate to high reliability; and above 0.9, high reliability (HAIR et al., 2009). However, values > 0.95 may indicate that the instrument contains many items that are assessing the same underlying concept. Thus, it suggests a high level of items with redundancy, where essentially the same item is rephrased in several different ways (SCHOLTES et al., 2011). It is therefore possible to state that the questions within the sub-scales clearly reflected the topic they addressed, indicating sufficient homogeneity of all the items. The removal of any single question did not significantly alter the results found by Cronbach's alpha for each of the sub-scales analysed, demonstrating that there was no need to eliminate any question for the Brazilian version (CRONBACH, 1951; HAIR et al., 2009).

These results found for internal consistency are in agreement not only with the findings of the validation of the original HOS in English (0.96 in the ADL subscale and 0.95 in the Sport subscale) (MARTIN et al., 2006), but also with the validation of the German version (0.95 in the ADL subscale and 0.91 in the Sport subscale) (NAAL et al., 2011), 2006); but also with the validation work of the German (0.95 ADL subscale and 0.91 Sport subscale) (NAAL et al., 2011), Spanish (0.95 ADL subscale and 0.9 Sport subscale) (SEIJAS et al., 2014) and Korean (0.948 ADL subscale and 0.958 Sport subscale) versions (LEE et al., 2014).

The reliability of the Brazilian version of the HOS was verified by the intra-rater test-retest, i.e. each patient answering the same questionnaire alone, without help, at two different times over a 48-hour interval. This test-retest interval was based on two criteria: it had to be long enough to prevent patients from remembering their previous answers, but at the same time short enough to avoid any changes in the patients' clinical condition.

In the validation study of the German version of the HOS, only 33 patients took part in the test-retest reliability assessment and the median time interval between assessments was 10 days. The patients selected had undergone surgical treatment for femoroacetabular impingement (NAAL et al., 2011). The validation study of the Spanish version assessed 100 patients with symptomatic hip disease for at least six months who answered the test-retest 15 days before undergoing surgical treatment for hip arthroscopy (SEIJAS et al., 2014). The validation study of the Korean version assessed 60 patients who were to undergo hip arthroscopy and the time interval between the test-retest was between two and three weeks before surgery (LEE et al., 2014). What can be seen is that there is no consensus in the literature on the ideal time interval for the test-retest. Perhaps the time interval between the test-retest in these studies was not short enough to avoid changes in the patients' clinical condition. Furthermore, it is difficult to say that these patients remained without any therapeutic support during this time interval.

The Brazilian version of the HOS questionnaire showed excellent intra-rater test-retest reliability, with ICC results of 0.992 for the ADL subscale and 0.994 for the Sport subscale. An ICC between 0.4 and 0.75 is considered satisfactory, and an ICC > 0.75 is excellent (BARTKO, 1966). This analysis showed that for all the questionnaire sub-scales, when comparing the first and second application times, all the ICC values were greater than 0.9. This indicates excellent intra-rater test-retest reliability and demonstrates that the HOS questionnaire is reproducible.

Our results were similar to those found in a study assessing the reliability of the original HOS in English (0.98 for the ADL subscale and 0.92 for the Sport subscale) (MARTIN; PHILIPPON, 2008). There was also similarity in the values found in the German (0.94 for the ADL subscale and 0.89 for the Sport subscale) (NAAL et al., 2011); Spanish (0.95 for the ADL subscale and 0.94 for the Sport subscale) (SEIJAS et al., 2014); and Korean (0.946 for the ADL subscale and 0.929 for the Sport subscale) versions (LEE et al., 2014).

A linear regression curve of the Bland-Altman graph was determined to assess the presence of a proportional deviation. The Bland-Altman and agreement-survival graphs showed adequate agreement between the test-retest of the Brazilian version of the HOS, indicating only a small variance between the means, with no statistically significant differences, as demonstrated by the results of the paired Student's t-test. The fixed bias shown in the linear regression curve increases reliability because, unlike a measure with proportional bias, the level of agreement with the HOS test-retest remained constant for the patients (ALTMAN; BLAND, 1983; BLAND; ALTMAN, 1986; LUIZ et al., 2003). The paired Student's t-test showed no statistically significant differences between the test-retest values ($p = 0.84$ for the ADL subscales and $p = 0.82$ for the Sport subscales) (VIEIRA, 2010).

In the Brazilian version of the HOS, the EPM found in the ADL subscale was 1.7 points, while in the Sport subscale it was 1.9 points. The DCM calculated was 4.6 points for the ADL subscale and 5.3 points for the Sport subscale (BARTLETT; FROST, 2008; SCHOLTES et al., 2011). In the reliability study of the original HOS in English, the DCM values were based on a 95% Confidence Interval of ± 3 points for both the ADL and Sports subscales (MARTIN; PHILIPPON, 2008). In the study of the German version of the HOS, the EPM was ± 4 (95% CI, 3 to 6 points) for the ADL subscale and ± 8 (95% CI, 6 to 11 points) for the Sport subscale. In this same study, the DCM for the ADL subscale was 11 points and for the Sport subscale it was 22 points (NAAL et al., 2011). In the Spanish version, the EPM was ± 5.1 for ADL and ± 8.5 for Sport; and the MCD was 13.7 points for the ADL subscale and 22.8 points for the Sport subscale (SEIJAS et al., 2014). However, in the study of the Korean version, no evidence was found to analyse these measures (LEE et al., 2014). Perhaps the discrepancy between the results of this study and other validation studies is due to the excessively long test-retest interval.

Knowing the amount of measurement error contributes to assessing the outcome of surgeries or other treatments performed, and indicates whether relevant clinical changes have occurred in the patient (SCHOLTES et al., 2011; MOKKINK et al., 2016). The concordance-survival graphs for the Brazilian version of the HOS suggest that values above 7 points for the ADL subscale and 6 points for the Sport subscale represent the amount of change in the score needed to be considered greater than the measurement error and represent a real change in the patient's health condition.

In this study, construct validity was tested by comparing the Brazilian version of the HOS with the NAHS and SF-12 questionnaires - which have already been validated for Brazilian Portuguese - using Pearson's correlation coefficient. Analysing the convergent construct validity between the ADL subscale of the Brazilian version of the HOS and the

NAHS questionnaire showed a strong correlation: 0.874. The same occurred with the correlation between the Sports subscale of the HOS and the Physical subscale of the SF-12: 0.744. There was also a strong correlation between the Sport subscale of the HOS and the NAHS questionnaire: 0.789. There was a moderate correlation between the Sport subscale of the HOS and the Physical subscale of the SF-12: 0.685. After verifying the existence of a strong, moderate and significant correlation between the ADL and Sport subscales of the HOS with the NAHS questionnaire and the Physical subscale of the SF-12, it is possible to interpret that the scores of the HOS subscales converge with the scores of the other questionnaires analysed. The higher correlation values between the HOS and the NAHS showed that the two instruments had similar characteristics. This can be explained by the fact that the NAHS is also a hip-specific instrument and has questions that address pain, mechanical symptoms, function and physical activity - whereas the SF-12 is a generic quality of life questionnaire (VIEIRA, 2010).

The analysis of divergent construct validity between the ADL and Sport subscales of the Brazilian version of the HOS and the Mental subscale of the SF-12 obtained values of 0.346 and 0.344, respectively. There were weak and non-significant correlations between the sub-scales analysed. In this case, it is possible to conclude that there is a divergence between the scores tested when considering the HOS ADL and Sports subscales and the SF-12 Mental subscale. Thus, it was possible to consider the HOS questionnaire as converging and diverging appropriately in relation to the proposed construct (VIEIRA, 2010).

In the validation study of the German version of the HOS (NAAL et al., 2011), there was a strong correlation between the HOS subscales and the Physical subscale of the SF-12, but there was a weak correlation between the HOS subscales and the Mental subscale of the SF-12 - similar to the Brazilian study. Similar results were also found in the validation study of the original HOS in English (MARTIN et al., 2006) and in the study of the Korean version of the HOS (LEE et al., 2014), which assessed the correlation of the HOS with the SF-36. In these studies, convergent construct validity was observed through the strong correlations between the HOS subscales and the SF-36 Physical subscale. In this case, the Mental Health subscale of the SF-36 had a weak correlation with the HOS subscales.

The Brazilian version of the HOS showed good content validity, as there was no evidence of questionnaires with the floor effect and/or ceiling effect. This result was similar to that found in the validation study of the Korean version (LEE et al., 2014). However, this finding differs from the results found in studies of the German and Spanish versions, which showed the presence of floor effect or ceiling effect (NAAL et al., 2011; SEIJAS et al., 2014).

Criterion validity is determined by the degree to which the scores of an instrument show themselves to be an adequate reflection of an instrument classified as the "gold standard". This property was not assessed in this study because, according to the group that developed COSMIN, there is no health assessment instrument that is classified as a "gold standard" (MOKKINK et al., 2010b; SCHOLTES et al., 2011; MOKKINK et al., 2016). Therefore, the validity of the Brazilian version of the HOS was determined by the psychometric properties of construct validity and content validity.

The validation studies of the Spanish (SEIJAS et al., 2014) and Korean (LEE et al., 2014) versions of the HOS assessed responsiveness in patients who underwent surgical treatment six months after surgery. The study of the Brazilian version of the HOS did not assess this psychometric property, as we did not reapply the questionnaire to patients after a long period of time. However, the absence of this analysis did not prevent the validation of the Brazilian version of the HOS. Further studies are underway to assess the responsiveness of this questionnaire.

This lack of prospective re-evaluation of the patients was a limitation of this study, which did not assess the change in quality of life after treatment, due to the lack of patient compliance. Another limitation was the fact that all the patients were selected from a single centre belonging to the private health network in Rio de Janeiro and the results found may not correspond to the reality of the Brazilian population.

CHAPTER 7

CONCLUSION

The Brazilian version of the Hip Outcome Score (HOS-Brasil) questionnaire was validated in a group of physically active patients with a medical diagnosis of femoroacetabular impingement or peritrochanteric pain syndrome.

The psychometric properties of reliability and validity showed excellent internal consistency, intra-rater test-retest reliability, content validity and construct validity. The measurement error indicated that values above 7 points for the ADL subscale and 6 points for the Sport subscale represent a real change in the patient's health condition. Further studies are underway to assess the responsiveness of the Brazilian version of the Hip Outcome Score.

The process of validating the Brazilian version of the Hip Outcome Score questionnaire made this quality of life assessment tool valid and reliable for the Brazilian Portuguese language and will thus provide doctors and health professionals in Brazil with an instrument capable of assessing physically active patients with hip diseases without serious degenerative changes.

REFERENCES

ALTMAN, D. G.; BLAND, J. M. Measurement in medicine: the analysis of method comparison studies. Statistician, 1983; 32:207-17.

BARTKO, J. J. The Intraclass Correlation Coefficient as a Measure of Reliability. Psychological Reports, 1966; 19:3-11.

BARTLETT, J. W.; FROST, C. Reliability, repeatability and reproducibility: analysis of measurement errors in continuous variables. Ultrasound Obstet Gynecol, 2008; 31:466-75.

BEATON, D. E.; BOMBARDIE, C.; GUILLEMIN, F.; FERRAZ, M. B. Guidelines for the process of cross-cultural adaptation of self-report measures. Spine, 2000; 25(24):3186-91.

BELLAMY, N.; BUCHANAN, W. W.; GOLDSMITH, C. H.; CAMPBELL, J.; STITT, L. W. Validation study of WOMAC: A health status instrument for measuring clinically important patient relevant outcomes to antirheumatic drug therapy in patients with osteoarthritis of the hip or knee. J Rheumatol, 1988a; 15:1833-40.

______.; et. al. Validation study of WOMAC: A health status measure for measuring clinically important patient relevant outcomes following total hip or knee arthroplasty in osteoarthritis. J Orthop Rheumatol, 1988b; 1:95-108.

BLAND, J. M.; ALTMAN, D. G. Statistical methods of assessing agreement between two methods of clinical measurement. Lancet, 1986; 1:307-10.

BYRD, J. W. T. Avoiding the labrum in hip arthroscopy. Arthroscopy, 2000; 16:770- 3.

CAMELIER, A. A. Avaliação da qualidade de vida relacionada à saúde em pacientes com DPOC: estudo de base populacional com o SF-12 na cidade de São Paulo-SP [thesis]. São Paulo: Federal University of the State of São Paulo; 2004.

CHRISTENSEN, C. P.; ALTHAUSEN, P. L.; MITTLEMAN, M. A.; LEE, J. A.; MCCARTHY, J. C. The nonarthritic hip score: reliable and validated. Clin Orthop Relat Res, 2003; 406:75-83.

CICONELLI, R. M. Quality of life assessment measures. Rev Bras Reumatol, 2003; 43(2): 9-13.

CICONELLI, R. M.; FERRAZ, M.; SANTOS, W.; MEINÃO, I.; QUARESMA, M. Translation into Portuguese and validation of the generic quality of life assessment questionnaire SF-36 (Brazil SF-36). Rev Bras Reumatol, 1999; 39(3):143-50.

COIMBRA, I. B.; PASTOR, E. H.; GREVE, J. M. D. A.; PUCCINELLI, M. L. C.; FULLER, R.; CAVALCANTI, F. S.; MACIEL, F. M. B.; HONDA, E. Brazilian Consensus for the Treatment of Osteoarthritis (Osteoarthrosis) Rev Bras Reumatol, 2002; 42(6):371-4.

CROFT, P.; COOPE, R. C.; WICKHAM, C.; COGGON, D. Defining osteoarthritis of the hip for epidemiologic studies. Am J Epidemiol, 1990; 132(3):514-22.

CRONBACH, L. J. Coefficient alpha and internal structure of tests. Psichometrika, 1951; 16:297-334.

D'AUBIGNÉ, R. M.; POSTEL, M. Functional results of hip arthroplasty with acrylic prosthesis. J Bone Joint Surg Am, 1954; 36:451-75.

DAWSON, J.; FITZPATRICK, R.; CARR, A.; MURRAY, D. W. Questionnaire on the perception of patients about total hip replacement. J Bone Joint Surg Br, 1996; 78(2):185-90.

DEL CASTILLO, L. N.; LEPORACE, G.; CARDINOT, T. M.; LEVY, R. A.; OLIVEIRA, L. P. The *importance of questionnaires for assessing quality of life.* Rev Hosp Univ Pedro Ernesto, 2012; 11(1): 12-7.

DEL CASTILLO, L. N.; LEPORACE, G.; CARDINOT, T. M.; LEVY, R. A.; OLIVEIRA, L. P. *Translation, cross-cultural adaptation and validation of the Brazilian version of the Nonarthritic Hip Score.* São Paulo Med J, 2013; 131(4):244- 51.

ESCOBAR, A.; QUINTANA, J. M.; BILBAO, A.; AZKARATE, J.; GUENAGA, J. I. *Validation of the Spanish version of the WOMAC questionnaire for patients with hip or knee osteoarthritis.* Clin Rheumatol, 2002; 21:466-71.

EVERITT, B. S.; SKRONDAL, A. *The cambridge dictionary of statistics.* 4th ed. New York: Cambridge University Press, 2010.

FUJIKI, E. N.; FURLAN, C.; VALESIN FILHO, E. S.; SOUTELLO, H. P. F.; YAMAGUSHI, E. N. *Peritrochanteric bursitis:* description of a new semiological manoeuvre to aid diagnosis. Acta Ortop Bras, 2008; 16(5):296-300.

GANDEK, B.; WARE, J. E.; AARONSON, N. K.; APOLONE, G.; BJORNER, J. B.; BRAZIER, J. E.; BULLINGER, M.; KAASA, S.; LEPLEGE, A.; PRIETO, L.; SULLIVAN, M. Cross-Validation of Item Selection and Scoring for the SF-12 Health Survey in Nine Countries: Results from the IQOLA Project. J Clin Epidemiol, 1998; 51(11):1171-78.

GANZ, R.; LEUNIG, M.; LEUNIG-GANZ, K.; HARRIS, W. H. The etiology of osteoarthritis of the hip: an integrated mechanical concept. Clin Orthop Relat Res, 2008; 466(2):264-72.

GANZ, R.; PARVIZI, J.; BECK, M.; LEUNIG, M.; NÕTZLI, H.; SIEBENROCK, K. A. Femoroacetabular impingement: a cause for osteoarthritis of the hip. Clin Orthop Relat Res, 2003; 417:112-20.

GUILLEMIN, F.; BOMBARDIER, C.; BEATON, D. Cross-cultural adaptation of health-related quality of life measures: literature review and proposed guidelines. J Clin Epidemiol, 1993; 46(12):1417-32.

HAIR JR., J. F; ANDERSON, R.E.; TATHAM, R. L.; BLACK, W. C. Multivariate data analysis. 6. ed. Porto Alegre: Bookman, 2009.

HARRIS, W. H. Traumatic arthritis of the hip after dislocation and acetabular fractures: treatment by mould arthroplasty. J Bone Joint Surg Am, 1969; 51:737-55.

KLÀSSBO, M.; LARSSON, E.; MANNEVIK, E. *Hip disability and osteoarthritis outcome score.* An extension of the Western Ontario and McMaster Universities Osteoarthritis Index. Scand J Rheumatol, 2003; 32(1):46-51.

LEE, Y. K.; HA, Y. C.; MARTIN, R. L.; HWANG, D. S.; KOO, K. H. *Transcultural adaptation of the Korean version of the Hip Outcome Score.* Knee Surg Sports Traumatol Arthrosc, 2014.

LEQUESNE, M. G. *The algofunctional indices for hip and knee osteoarthritis.* J Rheumatol, 1997; 779-81.

LEUNIG, M.; BECK, M.; DORA, C.; GANZ, R. *Femoroacetabular impingement:* etiology and surgical concept. Oper Tech Orthop, 2005; 15:247-55.

LOPES, A. D.; CICONELLI, R. M.; REIS, F. B. *Measures for assessing quality of life and health status in orthopaedics*. Rev Bras Ortop, 2007; 42(11/12):355-9.

LUIZ, R. R.; COSTA, A. J. L.; KALE, P. L.; WERNECK, G. L. *Assessment of agreement of a quantitative variable:* a new graphical approach. J Clin Epidimiol, 2003; 56(10):963-7.

MARTIN, R. L. Hip arthroscopy and outcome assessment. Oper Tech Orthop, 2005; 15(3):290-96.

MARTIN, R. L.; KELLY, B. T.; PHILIPPON, M. J. Evidence of validity for the hip outcome score. Arthroscopy, 2006; 22(12):1304-11.

MARTIN, R. L.; PHILIPPON, M. J. Evidence of reliability and responsiveness for the hip outcome score. Arthroscopy, 2008; 24(6):676-82.

MARTIN, R. L.; PHILIPPON, M. J. Evidence of validity for the hip outcome score in hip arthroscopy. Arthroscopy, 2007; 23(8):822-26

MOHTADI, N. G.; GRIFFIN, D. R.; PEDERSEN, M. E.; CHAN, D.; SAFRAN, M. R. The Development and validation of a self-administered quality-of-life outcome measure for young, active patients with symptomatic hip disease: the International Hip Outcome Tool (iHOT-33). Arthroscopy, 2012; 28(5):595-605.

MOKKINK, L. B.; PRINSEN, C. A. C.; BOUTER, L. M.; DE VET, H. C. W.; TERWEE, C. B. The COnsensus-based Standards for the selection of health Measurement Instruments (COSMIN) and how to select an outcome measurement instrument. Braz J Phys Ther, 2016; 20(2):105-13.

MOKKINK, L. B.; TERWEE, C. B.; KNOL, D. L.; STRATFORD, P. W.; ALONSO, J.; PATRICK, D. L.; BOUTER, L. M.; DE VET, H. C. W. Protocol of the COSMIN study: COnsensus-based Standards for the selection of health Measurement Instruments. BMC Med Res Methodol, 2006; 6:2.

MOKKINK, L. B.; TERWEE, C. B.; KNOL, D. L.; STRATFORD, P. W.; ALONSO, J.; PATRICK, D. L.; BOUTER, L. M.; DE VET, H. C. W. The COSMIN checklist for evaluating the methodological quality of studies on measurement properties: A clarification of its content. BMC Med Res Methodol, 2010a; 10:22.

MOKKINK, L. B.; TERWEE, C. B.; PATRICK, D. L.; ALONSO, J.; STRATFORD, P. W.; KNOL, D. L.; BOUTER, L. M.; DE VET, H. C. W. The COSMIN study reached international consensus on taxonomy, terminology, and definitions of measurement properties for health-related patient-reported outcomes. J Clin Epidemiol, 2010b; 63:737-45.

NAAL, F. D.; IMPELLIZZERI, F. M.; MIOZZARI, H. H.; MANNION, A. F.; LEUNIG, M. The *German Hip Outcome Score:* validation in patients undergoing surgical treatment for femoroacetabular impingement. Arthroscopy, 2011; 27(3):339- 45.

NAAL, F. D.; MIOZZARI, H. H.; KELLY, B. T.; MAGENNIS, E. M.; LEUNIG, M.; NOETZLI, H. P. The Hip Sports Activity Scale (HSAS) for patients with femoroacetabular impingement. Hip Int, 2013; 23(2):204-11.

NEPPLE, J. J.; LEHMANN, C. L.; ROSS, J. R.; SCHOENECKER, P. L.; CLOHISY, J. C. Coxa profunda is not a useful radiographic parameter for diagnosing pincer-type femoroacetabular impingement. J Bone Joint Surg Am, 2013; 95(5):417-23.

NILSDOTTER, A. K.; LOHMANDER, L. S.; KLÀSSBO, M.; ROOS, E. M. *Hip disability and osteoarthritis outcome score (HOOS)* - validity and responsiveness in total hip replacement. BMC Musculoskelet Disord, 2003; 4:10.

OLIVEIRA, L. P.; CARDINOT, T. M.; DEL CASTILLO, L. N. C.; QUEIROZ, M. C.; POLESELLO, G. C. *Translation and cultural adaptation of the Hip Outcome Score to the Portuguese language*. Rev Bras Ortop, 2014; 49(3):297-304.

RAT, A. C.; COSTE, J.; POUCHOT, J.; BAUMANN, M.; SPITZ, E.; RETEL- RUDE, N.; QUINTREC, J. S. L.; DUMONT-FISCHER, D.; GUILLEMIN, F. *OAKHQOL:* A new instrument to measure quality of life in knee and hip osteoarthritis. J Clin Epidemiol, 2005; 58:47-55.

SAFRAN, M. R.; HARIRI, S. *Hip arthroscopy assessment tools and outcomes*. Oper Tech Orthop, 2010; 20(4):264-77.

SCHOLTES, V. A.; TERWEE, C. B.; POOLMAN, R. W. *What makes a measurement instrument valid and reliable?* Injury, Int. J. Care Injured, 2011; 42:236-40.

SEIJAS, R.; SALLENT, A.; RUIZ-IBÁN, M. A.; ARES, O.; MARÍN-PENA, O.; CUÉLLAR, R.; MURIEL, A. *Validation of the Spanish version of the hip outcome score*: a multicentre study. Health Qual Life Outcomes, 2014; 12:70.

SILVEIRA, M. F.; ALMEIDA, J. C.; FREIRE, R. S.; HAIKAL, D. S.; MARTINS, A. E. B. L. *Psychometric properties of the quality of life assessment instrument:* 12-item health survey (SF-12). Ciênc saúde coletiva, 2013; 18(7):1923-31.

THORBORG, K.; HOLMICH, P.; CHRISTENSEN, R.; PETERSEN, J.; ROOS, E. M. *The Copenhagen Hip and Groin Outcome Score (HAGOS):* development and validation according to the COSMIN checklist. J Sports Med Br, 2011; 45(6):478-91.

THORBORG, K.; ROOS, E. M.; BARTELS, E. M.; PETERSEN, J.; HOLMICH, P. *Validity, reliability and responsiveness of patient-reported outcome questionnaires when assessing hip and groin disability*: a systematic review. J Sports Med Br, 2010; 44(16):1186-96.

VIEIRA, S. Biostatistics: advanced topics. 3. ed. Rio de Janeiro: Elsevier, 2010.

WARE, J. E.; KOSINSKI, M.; KELLER, S. D. A 12-Item Short-Form Health Survey:

Construction of scales and preliminary tests of reliability and validity. Med Care, 1996; 34(3):220-33.

WARE, J. E.; SHERBOURNE, C. D. The MOS 36-item short-form health survey (SF-36). I. Conceptual framework and item selection. Med Care, 1992; 30(6):473-83.

WILLIAMS, B. S.; COHEN, S. P. Greater trochanteric pain syndrome: a review of anatomy, diagnosis and treatment. Anesth Analg, 2009; 108(5):1662-70.

APPENDIX A - Informed Consent Form

FREE AND INFORMED CONSENT FORM

The aim of this study was to validate the *Hip Outcome Score* (HOS) in Portuguese, which assesses quality of life in patients with hip disease.

This questionnaire will be of great importance as a functional assessment tool for patients with non-arthritic hip diseases and can be used as a way of informing patients about their state of health.

The *Hip Outcome Score is* made up of twenty-eight items divided into two subscales, nineteen items on activities of daily living (ADLs) and nine items on sports activities.

The questionnaire will be completed at two different times: on the first day, the *Hip Outcome Score* (HOS) will be completed together with the *Nonarthritic Hip Score* (NAHS) and the *12-item Short-Form Health Survey* (SF-12), and on the *second* day, after a 48-hour break, only the *Hip Outcome Score* (HOS) will be completed.

The study was approved by the Research Ethics Committee of the Pedro Ernesto University Hospital of the State University of Rio de Janeiro (HUPE-UERJ) under CEP/HUPE number 2674. The procedures adopted did not present any discomfort or risk and were non-invasive.

The researchers are available to answer any questions that may arise during or after the course of this study. If you have any further questions, please contact the coordinators.

All participants in the study are volunteers, so anyone can refuse to take part or withdraw their consent at any time.

The research team undertakes to keep all the information collected confidential. This information can only be used by the project team to intervene positively with the participant. The researchers may use the data collected, provided that the identity of the volunteers evaluated is fully protected.

By this instrument, which fulfils the legal requirements, Mr. (a)............................ bearer
identity card.., signs their Free and
Informed consent to take part in the proposed research. And because they agree, they sign this agreement.

Rio de Janeiro,de de.

Participant's signature

Rafaela Maria de Paula Costa - researcher

Liszt Palmeira de Oliveira - researcher

APPENDIX B - Identification and clinical assessment form

IDENTIFICAÇÃO E DADOS DEMOGRÁFICOS

Nº do registro no estudo__________ (não preencher)
Nº do registro/matrícula:______________ (não preencher)

Nome:
Data:
Data de nascimento: **Idade:** anos
Estado civil: ☐ Casado ☐ Solteiro ☐ Viúvo ☐ Outro ________
Endereço:
Telefones:
E-mail:
Naturalidade:

Escolaridade
Alfabetizado: ☐ não ☐ sim
Grau de escolaridade: ☐ 1º grau incompleto ☐ 1º grau completo
☐ 2º grau incompleto ☐ 2º grau completo
☐ 3º grau incompleto ☐ 3º grau completo
Profissão:

AVALIAÇÃO CLÍNICA

Tempo de doença (dos sintomas):
Quadril acometido: ☐ Esquerdo ☐ Direito ☐ Esquerdo e direito
Se responder "esquerdo e direito", qual dói mais? ☐ Esquerdo ☐ Direito

Atividade física: ☐ sim ☐ não
Qual?
Frequência semanal:
Tratamento anterior: ☐ sim ☐ não
Qual?
Tratamento atual: ☐ sim ☐ não
Qual?

Diagnóstico Médico:

APPENDIX C - Individual clinical characteristics of the 70 selected patients

Patient	Gender	Age	Medical Diagnosis
1	M	49	IFA
2	F	25	SDPT
3	M	20	IFA
4	M	59	IFA
5	F	37	SDPT
6	M	35	IFA
7	M	35	IFA
8	F	39	SDPT
9	M	65	IFA
10	F	44	SDPT
11	F	52	IFA
12	F	24	SDPT
13	F	25	SDPT
14	F	49	SDPT
15	M	40	IFA
16	F	29	SDPT
17	F	29	IFA
18	M	35	IFA
19	F	44	IFA
20	M	34	IFA
21	F	41	SDPT
22	F	25	SDPT
23	F	42	SDPT
24	F	48	SDPT
25	F	64	SDPT
26	M	26	IFA
27	M	52	IFA
28	M	56	IFA
29	M	25	IFA
30	M	28	IFA
31	F	44	SDPT
32	F	30	SDPT
33	M	36	IFA
34	F	52	SDPT
35	F	51	SDPT
36	F	19	SDPT
37	F	40	IFA
38	F	41	SDPT
39	F	54	SDPT
40	F	45	SDPT
41	F	55	SDPT
42	F	34	SDPT
43	F	45	SDPT
44	M	51	IFA
45	F	54	SDPT

46	F	38	SDPT
47	F	59	SDPT
48	F	50	SDPT
49	M	67	SDPT
50	F	70	SDPT
51	F	41	SDPT
52	F	55	SDPT
53	F	46	SDPT
54	F	31	SDPT
55	F	58	SDPT
56	F	59	SDPT
57	F	34	SDPT
58	M	28	IFA
59	M	38	IFA
60	M	38	IFA
61	M	33	IFA
62	F	30	SDPT
63	M	46	IFA
64	F	46	IFA E
65	M	46	SDPT
66	M	21	IFA
67	F	68	SDPT
68	F	56	SDPT
69	F	68	SDPT
70	F	55	SDPT

Key: Male (M); Female (F); Femoroacetabular impingement (FAI); Peritrochanteric pain syndrome (PTPS).
Source: The author, 2017.

ANNEX A - Ethics committee: research approval

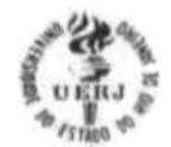

UNIVERSIDADE DO ESTADO DO RIO DE JANEIRO
HOSPITAL UNIVERSITÁRIO PEDRO ERNESTO
COMITÊ DE ÉTICA EM PESQUISA

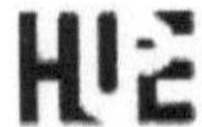

Rio de Janeiro, 21 de maio de 2010

Do: Comitê de Ética em Pesquisa
Prof.: Wille Oigman
Para: Prof. Bruno Tavares Rabello e Prof. Liszt Palmeira / Ortopedia

Registro CEP/HUPE: 2674 (este número deverá ser citado nas correspondências referentes ao projeto)
CAAE: 0119.0.228.000-10

O Comitê de Ética em Pesquisa do Hospital Universitário Pedro Ernesto, após avaliação, considerou o projeto, "TRADUÇÃO, ADAPTAÇÃO CULTURAL E VALIDAÇÃO DO HIP OUTCOME SCORE PARA A LÍNGUA PORTUGUESA" aprovado, encontrando-se este dentro dos padrões éticos da pesquisa em seres humanos, conforme Resolução n.º196 sobre pesquisa envolvendo seres humanos de 10 de outubro de 1996, do Conselho Nacional de Saúde.

O pesquisador deverá informar ao Comitê de Ética qualquer acontecimento ocorrido no decorrer da pesquisa.

O Comitê de Ética solicita a V. Sª., que ao término da pesquisa encaminhe a esta comissão um sumário dos resultados do projeto.

Prof. Wille Oigman
Presidente do Comitê de Ética em Pesquisa

CEP - COMITÊ DE ÉTICA EM PESQUISA
AV. VINTE E OITO DE SETEMBRO, 77 TÉRREO - VILA ISABEL - CEP 20551-030
TEL: 21 2587-6353 – FAX: 21 2264-0853 - E-mail: cep-hupe@uerj.br

ANNEX B - Ethics committee: approval of research extension

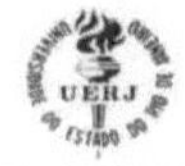

UNIVERSIDADE DO ESTADO DO RIO DE JANEIRO
HOSPITAL UNIVERSITÁRIO PEDRO ERNESTO
COMITÊ DE ÉTICA EM PESQUISA

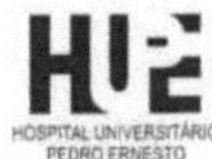

Rio de Janeiro, 19 de agosto de 2015

Do: Comitê de Ética em Pesquisa
Prof. Denizar Vianna Araújo
Para: Prof. Bruno Tavares Rabello e Prof. Liszt Palmeira / Ortopedia

Registro CEP/HUPE: 2674 (este número deverá ser citado nas correspondências referentes ao projeto)
CAAE: 0119.0.228.000-10

O Comitê de Ética em Pesquisa do Hospital Universitário Pedro Ernesto, após avaliação, considerou as considerações e justificativas para a prorrogação do projeto, "TRADUÇÃO, ADAPTAÇÃO CULTURAL E VALIDAÇÃO DO HIP OUTCOME SCORE PARA A LÍNGUA PORTUGUESA" aprovado, encontrando-se este dentro dos padrões éticos da pesquisa em seres humanos, conforme Resolução n.º466 sobre pesquisa envolvendo seres humanos de 12 de dezembro de 2012, do Conselho Nacional de Saúde, bem como o termo de consentimento livre e esclarecido.

O pesquisador deverá informar ao Comitê de Ética qualquer acontecimento ocorrido no decorrer da pesquisa.

O Comitê de Ética solicita a V. Sª., que ao término da pesquisa encaminhe a esta comissão um sumário dos resultados do projeto.

Prof. Denizar Vianna Araújo
Coordenador do Comitê de Ética em Pesquisa
COMITÊ DE ÉTICA EM PESQUISA
HUPE/UERJ

CEP - COMITÊ DE ÉTICA EM PESQUISA
AV. VINTE E OITO DE SETEMBRO, 77 TÉRREO - VILA ISABEL - CEP 20551-030
TEL: 21 2587-6353 – FAX: 21 2264-0853 - E-mail: cep-hupe@uerj.br

ANNEX C - Brazilian version of the *12-Item Short-Form* questionnaire

Health Survey (SF-12)

SF-12 quality of life questionnaire

INSTRUCTIONS: We want to know what you think about your health. This information will help us to know how you feel and how you are able to carry out your day-to-day activities. Please answer each question by ticking the appropriate box. If you are in doubt about how to answer the question, please reflect and just try to answer in the best way possible.

1. **In general, would you say that your health is: (tick one)**

2. ( ) excellent
3. ( ) very good
4. ( ) good
5. ( ) regular
6. ( ) bad

The following questions will deal with things that you do on average, in your day-to-day life (typical/ordinary day).

Do you think that your health now prevents you from doing some everyday things, for example:

2. Medium activities (such as moving a chair, shopping, cleaning the house, changing clothes)?

1. ( ) yes, it makes it very difficult
2. ( ) Yes, it's a bit difficult
3. ( ) No, it doesn't make it difficult at all

3. Do you think that your health now makes it difficult for you to carry out some everyday tasks, such as climbing three or more flights of stairs?

1. ( ) yes, it makes it very difficult
2. ( ) Yes, it's a bit difficult
3. ( ) No, it doesn't make it difficult at all

During the last 4 weeks, have you had any of the following problems with your work or day-to-day activities, for example:

4. Have you done less than you'd like because of your physical health?

1. ( ) yes
2. ( ) No

5. Have you had difficulty at work or in other activities because of your physical health?

1. ( ) yes
2. ( ) No

6. Have you done less than you would have liked because of emotional problems?

1. ( ) yes
2. ( ) No

7. Have you stopped doing your work or other activities as carefully as usual because of emotional problems?

1. ( ) yes
2. ( ) No

8. During the last 4 weeks, has any pain disrupted your normal work (both work at home and work outside the home)?

1. ( ) No, not at all
2. ( ) a little
3. ( ) moderately
4. ( ) a lot
5. ( ) extremely

These questions will look at how you feel and how things have been going for you over the last 4 weeks. For each question, please give the answer that most closely resembles the way you've been feeling.

How long during the last 4 weeks:

9. Did you feel calm and at ease?

1. ( ) all the time
2. ( ) most of the time
3. ( ) a good part of the time
4. ( ) some of the time
5. ( ) a small part of the time
6. ( ) Not a bit of the time

10. Did you have enough energy?

1. ( ) all the time
2. ( ) most of the time
3. ( ) a good part of the time
4. ( ) some of the time
5. ( ) a small part of the time
6. ( ) Not a bit of the time

11. Did you feel discouraged and depressed?

1. ( ) all the time
2. ( ) most of the time
3. ( ) a good part of the time
4. ( ) some of the time
5. ( ) a small part of the time
6. ( ) Not a bit of the time

12. During the last 4 weeks, how much of your time did your health or emotional problems get in the way of your social activities, such as visiting friends, relatives, going out, etc.?

1. ( ) all the time
2. ( ) most of the time
3. ( ) some of the time
4. ( ) a small part of the time
5. ( ) Not a bit of the time

ANNEX D - Brazilian version of the *Nonarthritic Hip Score* (NAHS) questionnaire

NONARTHRITIC HIP SCORE (NAHS) QUESTIONNAIRE

The following five questions assess the intensity of the pain you are feeling in the hip being assessed today. For each situation, please tick the answer that most accurately reflects the intensity of the pain felt in the last 48 hours.

How severe your pain is:

	None	Lightweight	Moderate	Strong	Very Strong
1 - Walking on flat ground					
2 - Going up or down stairs					
3 - At night, in bed					
4 - Sitting or lying down					

5 - Standing					

The following four questions refer to the symptoms you are experiencing in the hip being assessed today. For each situation, tick the answer that most accurately reflects the symptoms you have experienced in the last 48 hours.

How difficult you find it:

	None	Lightweight	Moderate	Strong	Very strong
1 - Locking or blocking your hip					
2 - Your hips moving out of place					
3 - Stiffness in your hip					
4 - Decreased movement in your hip					

The following five questions assess your physical condition. For each of these activities, tick the answer that most accurately reflects the difficulties you have experienced in the last 48 hours because of your hip.

How difficult is it for you?

	None	Lightweight	Moderate	Strong	Very strong
1 - Going down stairs					
2 - Climbing stairs					
3 - Getting up from a sitting position					
4 - Putting on socks					
5 - Getting out of bed					

The following six questions assess your ability to participate in certain types of activities. For each of the following activities, tick the answer that most accurately reflects the difficulty you have experienced in the last month because of pain in your hip. If you haven't taken part in a certain type of activity, imagine how much difficulty your hip could cause if you had done that activity.

How much difficulty your hip causes when you take part in:

	None	Lightweight	Moderate	Strong	Very strong
1 - High-intensity sports (e.g. football, judo, volleyball and aerobic exercise)					
2 - Low-intensity sports (for example, table tennis and bowling)					
3 - Running (as exercise)					
4 - Walking (as exercise)					

5 - Heavy domestic activities (e.g. moving furniture, cleaning, washing clothes in the sink)					
6 - Light domestic activities (e.g. cooking, dusting, washing up)					

ANNEX E - Brazilian version of the *Hip Outcome Score* questionnaire (HOS-Brazil)

HIP *OUTCOME SCORE* (HOS)

- ACTIVITIES OF DAILY LIVING SCALE (AVD):

Please answer all the questions with the option that best describes your conditions in the last week.

1. Stand for 15 minutes
( ) without difficulty
( ) Little difficulty
( ) Moderate difficulty
( ) extreme difficulty
( ) can't do it

2. Getting in and out of the car
( ) without difficulty
( ) Little difficulty
( ) Moderate difficulty
( ) extreme difficulty
( ) can't do it

3. Putting on socks and shoes
( ) without difficulty
( ) Little difficulty
( ) Moderate difficulty
( ) extreme difficulty
( ) can't do it

4. Climbing an inclined slope
( ) without difficulty
( ) Little difficulty
( ) Moderate difficulty
( ) extreme difficulty
( ) can't do it

5. Going down an incline
( ) without difficulty
( ) Little difficulty
( ) Moderate difficulty
( ) extreme difficulty
( ) can't do it

6. Climb a flight of stairs
( ) without difficulty
( ) Little difficulty
( ) Moderate difficulty
( ) extreme difficulty
( ) can't do it

7. Going down a flight of stairs
( ) without difficulty
( ) Little difficulty
( ) Moderate difficulty
( ) extreme difficulty
( ) can't do it

8. Getting on and off the kerb
( ) without difficulty
( ) Little difficulty
( ) Moderate difficulty
( ) extreme difficulty
( ) can't do it

9. Exaggerated squat
( ) without difficulty
( ) Little difficulty

10. getting in and out of the bath
( ) without difficulty
( ) Little difficulty

( ) Moderate difficulty
( ) extreme difficulty
( ) can't do it

( ) Moderate difficulty
( ) extreme difficulty
( ) can't do it

11. sit for 15 minutes

( ) without difficulty
( ) Little difficulty
( ) Moderate difficulty
( ) extreme difficulty
( ) can't do it

12.Start of the walk

( ) without difficulty
( ) Little difficulty
( ) Moderate difficulty
( ) extreme difficulty
( ) can't do it

13. walk for approximately 10 minutes

( ) without difficulty
( ) Little difficulty
( ) Moderate difficulty
( ) extreme difficulty
( ) can't do it

14. walking for 15 minutes or more

( ) without difficulty
( ) Little difficulty
( ) Moderate difficulty
( ) extreme difficulty
( ) can't do it

- Because of your hips, how much difficulty do you have in..:

15. turning on the affected leg

( ) without difficulty
( ) Little difficulty
( ) Moderate difficulty
( ) extreme difficulty
( ) can't do it

16. turning over in bed

( ) without difficulty
( ) Little difficulty
( ) Moderate difficulty
( ) extreme difficulty
( ) can't do it

17. light to moderate work (standing and walking)

( ) without difficulty
( ) Little difficulty
( ) Moderate difficulty
( ) extreme difficulty
( ) can't do it

18 Heavy work (pushing/pulling/climbing/loading)

( ) without difficulty
( ) Little difficulty
( ) Moderate difficulty
( ) extreme difficulty
( ) can't do it

19 Recreational activities

( ) without difficulty
( ) Little difficulty
( ) Moderate difficulty
( ) extreme difficulty
( ) can't do it

20.How would you quantify your level of function during the usual activities of daily living from 0 to 100, with 100 being your level of function before your hip problem and 0 being the impossibility of carrying out your usual activities of daily living.

0 10 20 30 40 50 60 70 80 90 100

- SPORTS SCHEDULE:

Because of your hips, how difficult it is for you:

1. Run 1.5 kilometres
( ) without difficulty
( ) Little difficulty
( ) Moderate difficulty
( ) extreme difficulty
( ) can't do it

2. Skip
( ) without difficulty
( ) Little difficulty
( ) Moderate difficulty
( ) extreme difficulty
( ) can't do it

3. Swinging objects, like in a golf swing
( ) without difficulty
( ) Little difficulty
( ) Moderate difficulty
( ) extreme difficulty
( ) can't do it

4. Landing on the ground after jumping
( ) without difficulty
( ) Little difficulty
( ) Moderate difficulty
( ) extreme difficulty
( ) can't do it

5. Start and stop quickly
( ) without difficulty
( ) Little difficulty
( ) Moderate difficulty
( ) extreme difficulty
( ) can't do it

6. Sudden change of direction / Lateral movements
( ) without difficulty
( ) Little difficulty
( ) Moderate difficulty
( ) extreme difficulty
( ) can't do it

7. Low-impact activities, such as brisk walking
( ) without difficulty
( ) Little difficulty
( ) Moderate difficulty
( ) extreme difficulty
( ) can't do it

8. Ability to carry out activities with normal technique
( ) without difficulty
( ) Little difficulty
( ) Moderate difficulty
( ) extreme difficulty
( ) can't do it

9. Ability to participate in your desired sport for as long as you'd like
( ) without difficulty
( ) Little difficulty
( ) Moderate difficulty
( ) extreme difficulty
( ) can't do it

10. How would you quantify your functional level during sporting activities, ranging from 0 to 100, with 100 being the level of function in these activities before the hip

problem and 0 being the impossibility of carrying out the sporting activities that were carried out before.

____

0 10 20 30 40 50 60 70 80 90 100

11. How do you quantify your current functional level?

( ) Normal
( ) Almost normal
( ) Abnormal
( ) Very abnormal

ANNEX F - *Hip Outcome Score* (HOS) Questionnaire: original in English

HIP OUTCOME SCORE (HOS)

Please answer **<u>every question</u>** with <u>one response</u> that most closely describes to your condition within the past week.
If the activity in question is limited by something other than your hip mark <u>not applicable (N/A)</u>.

Activities of Daily Living subscale

	No difficulty at all	Slight difficulty	Moderate difficulty	Extreme difficulty	Unable to do	N/A
Standing for 15 minutes	☐	☐	☐	☐	☐	☐
Getting into and out of an average car	☐	☐	☐	☐	☐	☐
Putting on socks and shoes	☐	☐	☐	☐	☐	☐
Walking up steep hills	☐	☐	☐	☐	☐	☐
Walking down steep hills	☐	☐	☐	☐	☐	☐
Going up 1 flight of stairs	☐	☐	☐	☐	☐	☐
Going down 1 flight of stairs	☐	☐	☐	☐	☐	☐
Stepping up and down curbs	☐	☐	☐	☐	☐	☐
Deep squatting	☐	☐	☐	☐	☐	☐
Getting into and out of a bath tub	☐	☐	☐	☐	☐	☐
Sitting for 15 minutes	☐	☐	☐	☐	☐	☐
Walking initially	☐	☐	☐	☐	☐	☐
Walking approximately 10 minutes	☐	☐	☐	☐	☐	☐
Walking 15 minutes or greater	☐	☐	☐	☐	☐	☐

Because of your hip how much difficulty do you have with:

	No difficulty at all	Slight difficulty	Moderate difficulty	Extreme difficulty	Unable to do	N/A
Twisting/pivoting on involved leg	☐	☐	☐	☐	☐	☐
Rolling over in bed	☐	☐	☐	☐	☐	☐
Light to moderate work (standing, walking)	☐	☐	☐	☐	☐	☐
Heavy work (push/pulling, climbing, carrying)	☐	☐	☐	☐	☐	☐
Recreational activities	☐	☐	☐	☐	☐	☐

How would you rate your current level of function during your usual activities of daily living from 0 to 100 with 100 being your level of function prior to your hip problem and 0 being the inability to perform any of your usual daily activities?

☐☐☐.0 %

Sports subscale

Because of your hip how much difficulty do you have with:

	No difficulty at all	Slight difficulty	Moderate difficulty	Extreme difficulty	Unable to do	N/A
Running one mile	☐	☐	☐	☐	☐	☐
Jumping	☐	☐	☐	☐	☐	☐
Swinging objects like a golf club	☐	☐	☐	☐	☐	☐
Landing	☐	☐	☐	☐	☐	☐
Starting and stopping quickly	☐	☐	☐	☐	☐	☐
Cutting/lateral movements	☐	☐	☐	☐	☐	☐
Low impact activities like fast walking	☐	☐	☐	☐	☐	☐
Ability to perform activity with your normal technique	☐	☐	☐	☐	☐	☐
Ability to participate in your desired sport as long as you would like	☐	☐	☐	☐	☐	☐

How would you rate your current level of function during your sports related activities from 0 to 100 with 100 being your level of function prior to your hip problem and 0 being the inability to perform any of your usual daily activities?

☐☐☐.0 %

How would you rate your current level of function?

☐ Normal ☐ Nearly normal ☐ Abnormal ☐ Severely abnormal

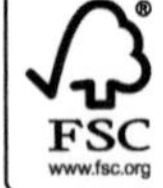

MIX
Papier aus verantwortungsvollen Quellen
Paper from responsible sources
FSC® C105338

Printed by Books on Demand GmbH, Norderstedt / Germany